FAC
Regia Medicorum et Chirurgorum
GLASGUENSIS.

Sciatis Virum Probum

David Collins

postquam Curriculum Disciplinarum nostris legibus statutum peregisset scientiam suam peritiamque nostro examine tam publico quam privato luculenter probasse et Nostram Licentiam plenissimam ad actus Chirurgiae et Pharmaceuticae omnes singulosque exercendos legitime consecutum fuisse.

Glasguae anno salutis humanae millesimo nongentesimo quadragesimo uno mensis Januarii die vicesimo quinto

Roy P. Young Praeses.

James W. MacDonald Inspector.

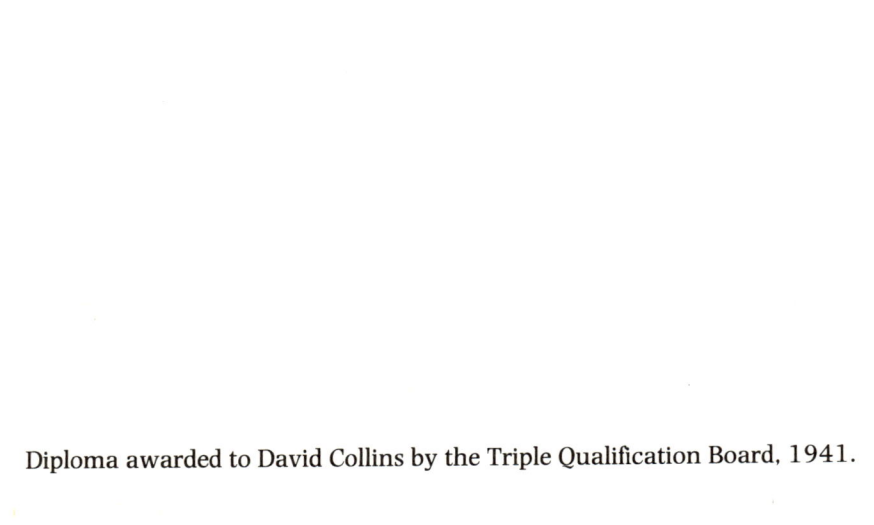

Diploma awarded to David Collins by the Triple Qualification Board, 1941.

GO AND LEARN

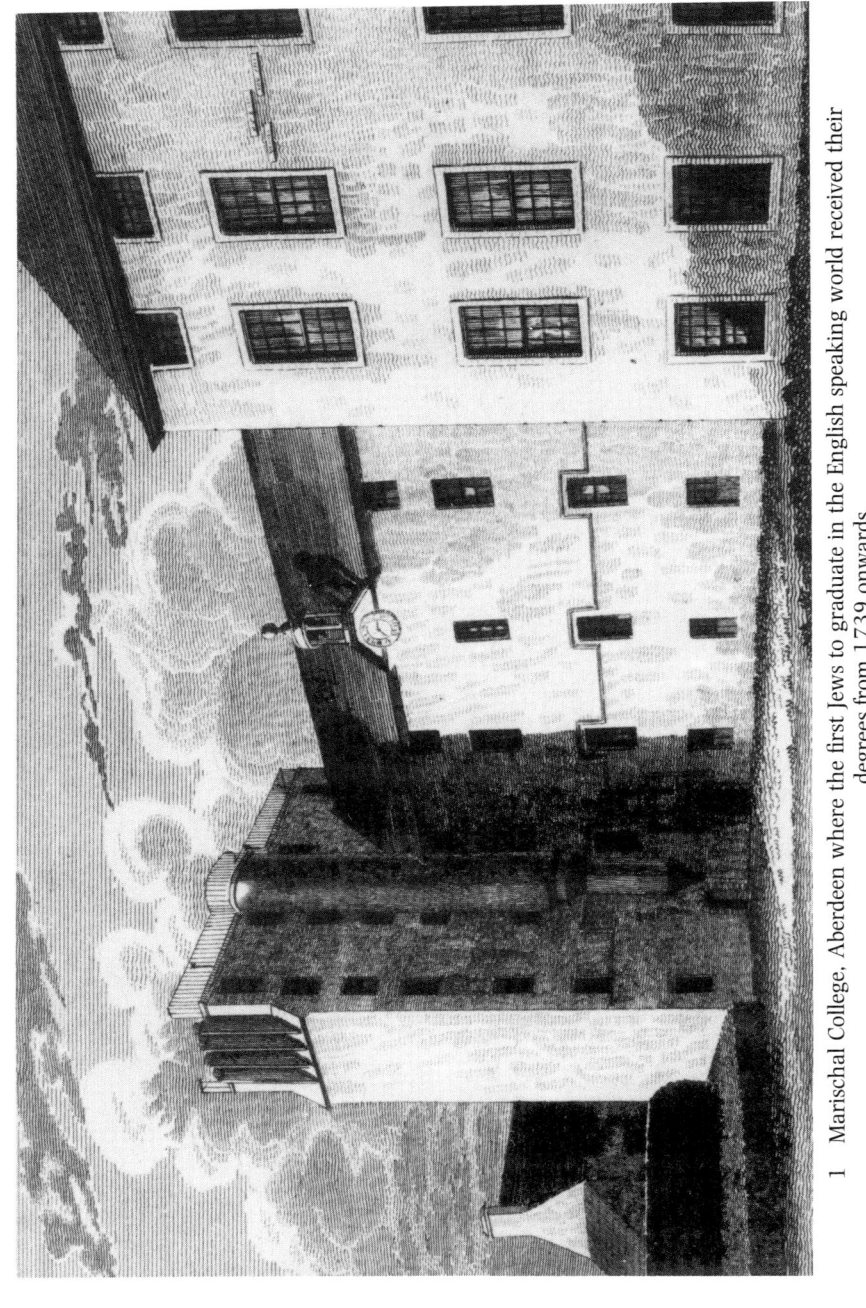

1 Marischal College, Aberdeen where the first Jews to graduate in the English speaking world received their degrees from 1739 onwards.

GO AND LEARN
the international story of Jews and Medicine in Scotland

KENNETH COLLINS

ABERDEEN UNIVERSITY PRESS

First published 1988
Aberdeen University Press
A member of the Pergamon Group

© Kenneth Collins 1988

British Library Cataloguing in Publication Data

Collins, Kenneth
  Go and learn.
  1. Scotland. Medicine. Role 1800-1945
  of Jews
  I. Title
  610'.8924

ISBN 0 08 036408-X

PRINTED IN GREAT BRITAIN
THE UNIVERSITY PRESS
ABERDEEEN

Dedicated to the memory of
Dr. David Collins (1912-1982) who saw the work begin
and of
Mr. Louis Ockrim (1896-1987) who lived to see it completed.

צֵא וּלְמַד

'Tza Ulmad' — 'Go and Learn' (Passover Hagadah)

Contents

LIST OF ILLUSTRATIONS		viii
ACKNOWLEDGEMENTS		x
ABBREVIATIONS		xii
INTRODUCTION		xiii
ONE	The Jewish Medical Tradition	1
TWO	Medicine and Education in Scotland	15
THREE	Jews in Medicine in Scotland before 1880 and the Development of the Immigrant Tradition	33
FOUR	The Growth and Development of Scottish Jewry	57
FIVE	The Movement of Jews into the Medical Profession in Scotland from 1880	81
SIX	American Jewish Medical Students in Scotland 1925–1940	98
SEVEN	European Refugee Physicians in Scotland 1933–1945	133
	Conclusion	159
APPENDICES		163
GLOSSARY		181
BIBLIOGRAPHY		182
INDEX		190

Acknowledgements

The researching of material for this work has involved my spending a considerable amount of time in various libraries in Scotland, England and the United States of America. I gratefully acknowledge the help and support of the following persons and institutions:

Universities and Medical Schools

Dr. R. Smart, Keeper of the Muniments, University of St. Andrews
Dr. Derek Dow, Archivist, Greater Glasgow Health Board, University Archives, University of Glasgow
Dr. J. L. Potter, Executive Dean of the Faculty of Medicine, University of Edinburgh
Colin MacLaren, Archivist, Aberdeen University Library
Lawrence Babbington, Librarian, Royal College of Physicians and Surgeons of Glasgow
Dorothy Wardle, Librarian, Royal College of Surgeons at Edinburgh
Special Collections Department, Edinburgh University Library
Adrian Allan, Assistant Archivist, University of Liverpool

Libraries and Learned Societies

Dr. Nathan Kaganoff, Librarian, American Jewish Historical Society, Brandais University, Waltham, Mass.
The Weiner Library, Devonshire Street, London.
Edgar Samuel, Jewish Historical Society of England.
Louise Rosenthal, Secretary, Australian Jewish Historical Society.
Liz Fraser, Secretary, Society for the Protection of Science and Learning.
Colin Harris, Principal Library Assistant, Bodleian Library, Oxford.
Morag Williams, Archivist, Dumfries and Galloway Health Board.
Harry Stalker, Murray Royal Hospital, Perth.
Caroline Hannaway, Editor, Bulletin of the History of Medicine, Baltimore, Md.
Howard Davies, Search Department, Public Records Office, Kew, London.

Trusts

I would like to acknowledge the support of the Carnegie Trust for the Universities of Scotland for a grant towards a visit to New York and to the Wellcome Trust for a travel grant for a visit to Boston and Washington. I am also grateful to the Carnegie Trust, the Walton Trust, the Goldberg Trust, the Scottish Society for the History of Medicine and Sir Emanuel Kaye for their support of the publication of this book.

I am indebted to members of the St. Andrews Medical Alumni of America and in particular to its President, Phil Kozinn of New York and to Herbert Goldberg of Washington D.C. I am also grateful for the advice and information received from other American graduates of the Scottish medical schools, especially Harold Klein, Sid Druce, Paul Steinlauf and Phil Reisman, and must also express my gratitude to many of the refugee physicians who do not wish to be individually identified.

I am grateful to have had the opportunity of presenting some of the preliminary findings at the Wellcome Unit for the History of Medicine in Oxford, the Society for the Social History of Medicine, the Scottish Society for the History of Medicine, the British Congress for the History of Medicine, the Jewish Historical Society of England and the Glasgow branch of the Young Jewish Leadership Institute.

Finally, I should like to thank Anne Crowther and Rick Trainor who supervised my Ph.D. thesis and who provided a regular and unfailing stream of constructive advice; my secretary Nanette Aitken who has typed the text; my mother for giving me the encouragement to start and continue with the project; my wife Irene, who has endured the past three years with good humour and practical support; and my children, Eve, Tamar, Rachel and David who have continued to live with the typewriter.

Abbreviations

AAC	Academic Assistance Council
AMA	American Medical Association
BMA	British Medical Association
BMJ	British Medical Journal
CCNY	City College, New York
Ch.M.	Master of Surgery
Ed. Edin	Edinburgh
EMS	Emergency Medical Service
FO	Foreign Office
FRCP	Fellow of the Royal College of Physicians
Glas.	Glasgow
GMC	General Medical Council
HO	Home Office
JAMA	Journal of the American Medical Association
LFPS	Licentiate of the Faculty of Physicians and Surgeons of Glasgow
Ll.D.	Doctor of Laws
LMSSA	Licentiate of the Medical Society of Surgeons and Apothecaries
LRCP&S	Licentiate of the Royal Colleges of Physicians and Surgeons of Edinburgh
LRCPI	Licentiate of the Royal College of Physicians of Ireland
LRCSI	Licentiate of the Royal College of Surgeons of Ireland
LRFPS	Licentiate of the Royal Faculty of Physicians and Surgeons of Glasgow
LSA	Licentiate of the Society of Apothecaries
M.B. Ch.B.	Bachelor of Medicine and Bachelor of Surgery
M.D.	Doctor of Medicine
MOH	Medical Officer of Health
MPU	Medical Practitioners' Union
MRCSE	Member of the Royal College of Surgeons of England
RAMC	Royal Army Medical Corps
St. A.	St. Andrews
SPSL	Society for the Protection of Science and Learning

Introduction

The attachment of Jews to the medical profession dates back to antiquity and has continued into modern times. Jews have been represented in most branches of medicine in a proportion far greater than their relative numbers in society, whether in Britain, America and most other countries where Jewish communities are to be found. This long association has led to the idealisation of medicine as one, and often the only, career choice suitable for the young Jew. These trends were already apparent, prior to Jewish emancipation in Western Europe in the late eighteenth and early nineteenth centuries, and reached their peak after the First World War when the children of the wave of emigration from Eastern Europe began to enter medical schools in their new lands.

This work will show both the depth of loyalty of generations of Jews to the medical profession and how the path of the achievement of these medical ambitions so often led to Scotland. The entry of Jews into the medical profession in Europe had often been restricted by the application of religious and social barriers which sought to isolate the Jew. However, for the Jew who was determined to enter the medical profession there was always a medical school somewhere which would enable the medical ambitions to be realised. In mediaeval times it was Padua which was the magnet and in the seventeenth and eighteenth centuries intending Jewish doctors were attracted to the Dutch universities. This study will show how the Scottish universities and medical schools adopted this role from the eighteenth century onwards and enabled over a thousand Jews to graduate over the next two centuries when difficulties were placed in their way in their countries of origin.

Thus, this work will bring together various strands which have not been considered as a unit before. While there have been recent studies of Scottish medicine[1] and Scottish education[2] as well as histories of the Jews in Britain[3] and in eighteenth century medicine[4] especially in London, no attempt has previously been made to consider the role of the Jews in medicine in Scotland from the first half of the eighteenth century. This study will draw on elements of all these component parts.

It will refute suggestions made that Jews were not well represented in medicine in Britain before the beginning of the nineteenth century or that Jews failed to take advantage of the opportunities afforded by the medical education available in Scotland, and particularly in Edinburgh.[5,6]

In Chapter One the question 'Why Medicine?' is posed and is answered by setting the history of the Jews and the medical profession into its historical context and places the modern movement of the Jews into the medical profession as part of the long chain of Jewish medical tradition. It will show that the practice of medicine had always been a respected Jewish calling and that the number of Jews entering medical schools was as high as the conditions of the time would allow. The medical ideal was fostered by such rabbi-physicians as Moses Maimonides who bestrode the two worlds of Jewish learning and medical practice and was to be an enduring inspiration to future generations of Jewish physicians.

As Jews began to settle in Britain from the middle of the seventeenth century, Jews seeking to study at university were faced with the restrictive policies of the ancient English universities which imposed religious tests requiring students or graduates to subscribe to the articles of the Church of England. By the middle of the nineteenth century increasing numbers of Jews especially from the wealthier families, were seeking to enter the professions.[7] In London the majority of professionals in 1883 were lawyers, a trend not followed in the provinces.[8]

The difficulties encountered by Jews in entering fields such as the army and the law ensured that the primary thrust of Jewish professional ambition was into medicine, which carried a higher status than teaching which was often perceived to be best alternative.[9] The gradual movement of Jews into professional life vindicated the belief that the Jew could enter society on the basis of equality of opportunity.

In Chapter Two I will show why it was in Scotland that the conditions were right for Jews to begin to enter the medical professions in Britain. The attractions of the Scottish medical schools, especially in Edinburgh, were well known and led to medical students being drawn to Scotland from all over Britain as well as from such overseas areas as North America, the West Indies and South Africa. In the eighteenth and early nineteenth centuries many of the Jewish doctors taking Scottish qualifications were newcomers to Britain fleeing from intolerance. During the nineteenth century there were increasing numbers of local Jewish students entering medicine and by the twentieth century the bulk of the overseas Jewish students were derived from the United States of America and from South Africa and the normal expectation was that, once qualified, the new medical graduates would return home.

The development of the Scottish medical schools will be seen in the context of the Scottish enlightenment when the issues in the universities were settled in favour of the secular interests enhancing the moves towards greater religious freedoms. The question of religious tests in the Scottish universities will be examined and it will be seen that these were not employed to restrict the entry of students on religious grounds.

To understand why it was Scotland which proved attractive to Jews seeking medical studies in the eighteenth and early nineteenth centuries it will be necessary to examine briefly those factors which thrust Scottish medicine into such prominence in the period. There were financial as well as educational and religious reasons for study in Scotland and this combination was to give Scotland a major role in medical training, and to give it an international quality. In addition, the nature of the Scottish educational system itself, of which the universities formed the peak, must be understood as being part of a framework which allowed entry in the professions for those from a lower stratum in society, difficult though it might be. A small number of gifted poorer children might succeed if given an unusual degree of support by parents and teachers, and this will help to explain the large entry of Jews into medicine in Scotland after the acculturation of the Eastern European Jews who flooded into Scotland after 1880.

In Chapter Three the position of the Jews in the Scottish universities before 1880 will be examined. In order to do this it was first necessary to establish a system for the identification of Jewish students and graduates in the Scottish universities during this period. I have used Jewish bibliographies and lists of Jewish physicians and checked these names against all the entries in the Scottish matriculation and graduation albums, some of which date back to the beginning of the eighteenth century. Many lists of Jews in Britain are available. They also include synagogue records, which for the Sephardi Jewish community at Bevis Marks in London, are quite complete.

There are always difficulties in identifying Jews merely by their names and I have usually sought some independent corroboration of their Jewishness from contemporary or later sources. Unfortunately, there are many instances where what might appear to be Jewish surnames are held by non-Jews and there has been a Jewish custom, which has accelerated with the acculturation of Jews into British society, for Jews to adopt names which are not typically Jewish.

There is the additional problem that not all the lists of Jews compiled in the past can be treated as being completely accurate. It is, for example, not difficult to find some names on such lists as 'Jews in Regular Freemasonry', *TJHSE*, XXV, (1977) and 'Wills and Letters of Administration' in *Anglo-Jewish Notabilities* (1949) which belonged to non-Jews. This can simply be done by identifying these names in other contexts where the probability of their being Jewish is low.*

My policy has been to include as Jews all those for whom corroborative evidence exists as to their Jewishness or Jewish origins. Conversely, I have eliminated those whose evidence of Jewish attachment is slight and contrary evidence appears stronger. It is always possible that sins of omission and commission will occur because this method of identifying Jewish names in the eighteenth and early nineteenth centuries can never be completely accurate. This may occasionally have meant an unwarranted omission but means that the data produced is likely to reflect under-counting rather than over-counting.

Having identified Jewish practitioners as accurately as possible, it will then be possible to move on to an assessment of the first Jewish doctors and consider their status in medicine both in the framework of the Jewish community and

---

*There are many examples of this. Morrise Alexander is listed in 'Wills and Letters of Administration' but is also mentioned in the *Matriculation Album of the University of Glasgow 1727-1858* as belonging to an old Glasgow merchant family. William Balmain, a member of an old landed Scottish family who achieved prominence in Australia, is listed in 'Jews in Regular Freemasonry'.

in the wider context also. The factors which have previously been identified as making Scotland such an attractive place for the study of medicine can now be seen in the context of the use made by Jews in the century and a half from the first Jewish medical graduation in Aberdeen in 1739 to the transformation of the Jewish community in Britain with the large scale immigration after 1880.

I will show how the tale linking Jews and medicine in Scotland began over two centuries ago with the awarding of degrees *in absentia** and quickly followed with the entry of Jews into regular undergraduate study at the University of Edinburgh. The subsequent careers of these graduates can be studied to find the degree of mobility obtained by these qualifications, whether into the professional elites or into careers in the provinces, army and colonial service and within the Jewish community itself. In addition, Jews were attracted to Scotland from North America, the West Indies and South Africa and the reasons for this will be seen in the context both of their Jewish communities and of the medical education in these areas.

During the nineteenth century with the slow but steady growth of the Jews in Scotland, I will show how Jews entered the medical profession from the first half of the nineteenth century. It was clear that the doors of the Scottish medical schools were open to Jews and despite the small size of the Jewish community by the 1850's there had been several Scottish Jews studying medicine both in Edinburgh and Glasgow. The first Jews in medicine in Scotland included members of the Ashenheim and Levenston families, as well as Asher Asher whose career in medicine served as an example to succeeding generations of Scottish Jews who identified with his combination of medical practice, Jewish scholarship and communal service. These developments, prior to 1880, helped to set the scene for increased Jewish penetration of the medical profession in the years ahead.

In Chapter Four I will examine the growth and development of Scottish Jewry, particularly in the context of the transformation of Scottish Jewry after 1880 as large numbers of Jews from Eastern Europe entered Scotland. The initial concerns of the immigrant Jews were to secure an economic base, develop the educational, welfare and social fabric of the Jewish community and to give the next generation the opportunities in life which they had been denied. The increasing identification of the medical profession as the ideal career choice, far above all other professions, will be seen in the context of the integration of the community into the Scottish cultural and educational environment and will show that the level of penetration of the medical profession by Scottish Jews was at a level fully ten times their proportion in the Scottish population. The history of the Jewish community in this period has been compiled with the aid of oral evidence from older members of the Glasgow and Edinburgh Jewish communities and supplemented by material

---

*The term *in absentia* is applied, in this work, to degrees awarded without prior study in that university.

from the *Jewish Chronicle* of London, which carried provincial news items from its earliest days* and the *Jewish Echo*, founded in Glasgow in 1928.

When the movement of Jews into Medicine in Scotland from 1880 is examined in Chapter Five the problem of identification of Jewish names is now much less. Lists of Jewish students successful in class examinations as well as of Jewish graduates and prize winners appeared in the *Jewish Chronicle* and *Jewish Echo* from the earliest days of both newspapers. In particular, the *Jewish Echo* lists are very complete and include American and South African Jews as well as members of the local community.

It is possible to have names corroborated by contemporary students and this method was employed with Americans and refugee practitioners in Scotland as well as with the native Scottish Jews. Graduate lists were shown to Jewish graduates of the various Scottish medical schools who were able to identify their Jewish colleagues. This method was used during the late 1930's to estimate the numbers of American Jews studying medicine abroad.[10] The problem of surname changing was also mitigated by the inclusion in the university records of both the original, and more identifiably Jewish surname, as well as the more anglicised name adopted.

I have been able to show how all the Jewish communities in Scotland, both small and large, were represented in this movement into medicine and how a large professional group was created in the community before the outbreak of the Second World War with most Jews in general practice and a few in hospital practice. Illustrations of some medical careers are given showing examples of penetration into the university with the appointment of a Jewish Regius Professor, as well as the careers of some hospital consultants and general practitioners.

Children of the East European immigrants were able to throw off the factors in their environment which had held back their parents' advancement and enter the Scottish universities in large numbers. Oral evidence and the use of obituaries from the *BMJ* as well as the use of the *Medical Directory* give the opportunity to define the career opportunities of the Jewish graduates and to assess their impact on medicine in Scotland and beyond.

By examination of the matriculation slips of students in the Medical Faculty at the University of Glasgow it has been possible to compare the social origins of the Jewish students with those of the non-Jewish medical students as the matriculation slips contain both the students' addresses and parental occupations.

The career choices and destinations of the Jewish graduates in Scotland will be examined to determine the advancement achieved. Medical emigration has always been a Scottish tradition and was by no means confined to the Jews. Scots-trained physicians were to be found all over the world, and Jewish graduates formed a small element of the Scottish medical diaspora from the eighteenth century onwards. That the Jews arrived early in the history of the Scottish medical schools may have assisted their later integration as would

---

*The *Jewish Chronicle* was founded in 1841.

the international character of Scottish medicine. The financial structure of the Scottish medical schools will also be considered for it was often the fees paid by student incomers which guaranteed the physical survival of these schools. Thus liberal attitudes can be interwoven with economic considerations.

After examination of the movement of local Jews into the medical profession in Scotland the next two chapters revert to the theme of the Scottish medical schools offering an educational haven to those facing difficulties or proscriptions at home.

In Chapter Six I will examine the question of the American Jews who came in large numbers to study medicine in Scotland after 1925 until numbers fell with the outbreak of the Second World War in 1939. It will be seen that, as amongst Scottish Jews, there was a great desire within American Jewry for many of its sons to study medicine. The nature of the quota system which helped to exclude many Jews from certain of the American medical schools, particularly in the Eastern United States where there was the greatest concentration of American Jews, will be studied. This will show why so many American Jewish medical students went abroad in search of medical qualifications. Figures produced annually in the *JAMA* section on medical education and licensure shows that the reliance of American medical students overseas on the Scottish medical schools increased as the 1930's progressed. Why they arrived in such large numbers in Scotland can be seen in the light of conditions prevailing in the various medical schools.

Individual identification of American Jews was aided by the lists of Jewish students appearing in the *Jewish Echo* and by the corroboration by student contemporaries. This enabled the compilation of accurate lists of Jewish American students at the various Scottish medical schools and permitted comparison of the geographic origins of both Jewish and non-Jewish students from America who were studying medicine in Scotland.

I have relied heavily on oral evidence for information about the American Jewish medical students in Scotland. Questionnaires were sent to 120 American medical practitioners identified from the *American Medical Directory for 1982* as Scottish medical graduates for the period under consideration.* Replies were received from 41, a response rate of 34%, and eighteen of these were interviewed in New York, New Jersey and Washington D.C. which permitted the amplification of the material obtained from the questionnaire replies. The doctors interviewed gave much information on the medical and social life as encountered by the American students in the four Scottish cities.

About the same period, beginning in 1933 with the Nazi accession to power in Germany, thousands of refugees from Central Europe arrived in Britain, among whom were a number of qualified physicians. I will examine in Chapter Seven the obstacles put in the way of their obtaining British qualifications and will show how the Scottish Triple Qualification Board were prepared to step out of line with their English colleagues in making it easier for the

---

*See American Questionnaire in Appendix 2.

refugee doctors to requalify. The integration of the refugee physicians was not achieved without some dissension within the British medical profession and the numbers of practitioners admitted was restricted at the request of the BMA. Opposition to the refugees was not confined to such groups as the Medical Practitioners Union (MPU) but extended to Lord Dawson of Penn, President of the Royal College of Physicians of London. Dawson's attitudes to German Jewry, refugee doctors and the role of the Scottish colleges will be studied using primary contemporary sources. While the Scottish universities permitted a high enrolment of Scottish Jews as medical students their record of admitting overseas Jews fell short of that of the rapidly expanding extramural schools, where virtually all the refugee physicians studied and qualified.

It was well established during the 1930's that a substantial majority of the refugee physicians were Jewish. The number of non-Jewish doctors who left Germany on political grounds was small. This information was corroborated by information obtained from the questionnaire sent to refugee physicians.* These questionnaires were sent to 56 doctors, identified as being German graduates, who had obtained Scottish qualifications, from the *Medical Directory for 1986*. Replies were obtained from 41 practitioners, a response rate of 74%, and six of these were interviewed. This permitted the setting of the information about the refugee practitioners in a personal as well as professional and educational context. While the questionnaire found a small number of doctors who were not Jewish by religion they all admitted to being of Jewish parentage.

Further information on the American students and the Central European refugees was obtained by examination of the minute books of all the medical schools in Scotland. Comparison with the situation was made by examination of the records from several of the English medical schools. This information was supplemented by materials from such published minutes as those of the General Medical Council and the British Medical Association as well as by scrutinising primary archival material.

The common strand over the two centuries from 1739 to 1945 is that Jews were a constant feature in Scottish medicine. Their numbers depended on a large variety of external factors which will be discussed and analysed. Medicine was the Jewish, no less than the Scottish, obsession, and it was the combination of a number of fortuitous factors in Scottish education which permitted the realisation of the obsession for so many. That it was Scotland which offered the greatest opportunity to its Jewish community was no surprise. The door had been open to Jews, as well as other religious minorities, from the beginning of the eighteenth century, and Jews were among the first to take advantage of the Scottish system.

Scottish education managed to give the chance to at least some members of the poorer sections of society to advance. The lure of social advancement through medical qualification proved to be irresistible to Jews seeking to escape from the trap of poverty and traditional ghetto activities, whether in

---

*See European Questionnaire in Appendix 3.

Glasgow's Gorbals or in New York's Lower East Side. In the eighteenth and nineteenth centuries the Scottish medical schools flourished on the continued attraction of overseas students who included a number of Jews who could not obtain the qualifications elsewhere.

By the twentieth century Jewish concerns were different. The rise of Scottish Jewry and their increasing enrolment in medical studies ensured a continued Jewish presence in the Scottish medical schools. There was never any suggestion that there was any attempt to limit the number of Scottish Jews entering medical schools in Scotland. For the overseas Jewish medical students the situation was different, as the increasing demands of local medical students in the 1930's put greater pressure on the available university places. Nevertheless more than 100 American Jews and at least as many South African Jews entered the Scottish universities during the late 1920's and 1930's. It will be seen that a substantial proportion of the South African medical students in Scotland were Jewish. The South African Jews formed part of that large group of South Africans whose tradition of studying medicine in Scotland began in colonial times. The numbers of South Africans coming to Scotland only started to fall in the twentieth century with the rise of South African medical schools.

The entry of hundreds of refugee physicians from Central Europe threatened to channel many hundreds of doctors through any British medical institutions prepared to accept them. It was the flexibility of the Scottish medical schools and the willingness of the Scottish Triple Qualification Board which enabled over 340 refugee physicians to obtain their necessary British medical qualifications. While the universities were unable to provide the precise facilities required by the refugees, Scottish hospitals and extra-mural medical schools were able to continue the Scottish tradition of enabling outsiders to enter the medical profession.

Thus over two hundred years the Jewish medical experience in Scotland was a reflection of many of the wider issues in Jewish history. Scottish medicine had its Jewish entry from these fleeing the Inquisition in Portugal, from Nazi Germany and from the children of the refugees from Tsarist Russia. It also reflected the extent of the Jewish diaspora with Jews from the West Indies, from South Africa and Australia. Jewish graduates in Scotland formed a microcosm of Jewish society as a whole, embracing those like Asher Asher whose career brought together the worlds of Judaism and medicine and others for whom the university represented assimilation and the road out of the Jewish community.

Almost 1,500 Jews took Scottish qualifications in medicine in the two centuries after 1739 forging strong links between the Jewish and Scottish strands in medicine. Scottish medicine was able to accommodate this large group of Jews over a period of two hundred years for many different reasons. There was freedom from religious tests and an internationally recognised standard of teaching. By normal university standards Scottish university education was cheap and its medical schools generally required a high student enrolment for their economic wellbeing.

The Scottish educational system afforded the chance for the highly motivated and well supported 'lad o' pairts'. This tradition found a ready generation of Scots born Jews in the twentieth century who adopted the Scottish pattern of finding the opportunity for social advancement in medical qualification. The sons of the Gorbals tailors and pedlars entered medicine alongside the sons of the new Jewish bourgeoisie and of the rabbis and cantors of Scotland's synagogues. They confirmed that the Scottish democratic myth can best be understood in terms of the encouragement of a meritocratic tradition which laid great emphasis on the right of individuals to climb the social ladder.[11] This formed the basis of the movement of the growing Jewish professional element into the mainstream of Scottish and British professional life.

REFERENCES

1 David Hamilton, *The Healers* (Edinburgh 1982)
2 R. D. Anderson, *Education and Opportunity in Victorian Scotland* (Oxford 1983)
3 Harold Pollins, *Economic History of the Jews in England* (1982)
4 Richard Barnett, 'Dr. Jacob de Castro Sarmento and Sephardim in Medical Practice in 18th-Century London', *TJHSE* Vol. XXVII, pp.84-114
5 Entry on 'Medicine', *Jewish Encyclopaedia* (New York 1925) Vol. V111 p.419
6 Richard Barnett, 'Dr. Jacob de Castro Sarmento and Sephardim in Medical Practice in Eighteenth Century London', *TJHSE* (1982) p.113
7 Harold Pollins, op.cit., p.114
8 Joseph Jacobs, *Studies in Jewish Statistics, Social Vital and Anthropometric*, (1891) p.37
9 Geoffrey D. M. Block, 'Jewish Students at the Universities of Great Britain and Ireland—Excluding London', *The Sociological Review* 34 (1942), p.191
10 Jacob A. Goldberg, 'Jews in the Medical Profession', *Jewish Social Studies*, Vol. 1 (1939), p.332
11 Robert Anderson, 'Education and Society in Modern Scotland : A Comparative Perspective', *History of Education Quarterly* 25 (1985), p.478

ONE

The Jewish Medical Tradition

It has been said that for the Jewish people health has not been merely an aspiration but an obsession.[1] For members of a small minority struggling to achieve equality, the medical profession offered a route of entry into the mainstream of national life and an improvement in social status. It could also provide a safe and secure living.

Jews could be found in medicine, and in the European medical schools, as local conditions allowed. Jewish entry into the medical profession often ran parallel to the general attitudes to Jewish political and civic emancipation. However, to understand the continuing Jewish fascination with medicine and the close Jewish involvement in the medical profession from earliest times will require examination of the Jewish attitudes both to healing and to the role of the physician. In a world created by God the right of the physician to heal could not be taken for granted. After all, Jewish history contains groups like the Karaites, opponents of Rabbinic Judaism, who objected to medicine and healing. Their opposition was based on a literal interpretation of Exodus 16:26 which says that if the people keep the commandments of God, no disease will befall them for 'I am the Lord who healeth thee'.

The traditional Rabbinic view of this verse is different; Rashi* takes it to mean that God teaches man the commandments to save him from these diseases. The physician and codifier Maimonides (1135-1204) states in his commentary on the Mishna (Nedarim 4:4) that it is obligatory, from the Torah, for the physician to heal the sick.

The Shulchan Arukh† states (Yoreh Deah no.336) that the Torah gave the physician permission to heal. Moreover, it adds that this is a religious precept and is included in the category of saving life. If the physician withheld his services it is considered as if he had shed blood. The general Rabbinic attitude can be summarised as indicating that true healing is a gift from God who has given the physician the wherewithal to heal by natural means.

Ben Sira, in the Apocryphal book of Ecclesiasticus, expressed the Jewish attitude to the physician thus (Eccles.38):

> Honour a physician before need of him
> Him also has God apportioned
> From God a physician gets wisdom
> And from a King he shall receive gifts.

---

* Greatest of Bible exegetes, lived in 11th century France.
† Main codification of Jewish law, compiled in 16th century.

> The skill of a physician shall lift up his head
> And he shall stand before nobles
> God brings out medicines from the earth
> And let a prudent man not refuse them.

It is recommended in the Talmud (Sanhedrin 17b) that no wise person should reside in a town that does not have a physician and there are a large number of other Talmudic references to doctors and healing. Patients are required, not merely permitted, to seek medical help when required and all restrictions, such as those pertaining to the Sabbath may be set aside where there is any possible danger to life. The Talmud contains a large number of medical references, either from a small group of Rabbis who were also qualified to call themselves doctor, or pertaining to folk medicine and superstitions. Julius Preuss, who collected all the medical references in Jewish writings, suggests that the common maxim 'he who has pain should consult a physician' from Baba Kamma 46b in the Babylonian Talmud must be taken to mean that medical services would have been quite widespread upwards of 1,500 years ago.[2]

The 15th century Jewish philosopher Isaac Arama said that man must not rely on Providence alone or on miracles when it comes to healing and sickness.[3] It can be seen that there is ample evidence within the traditional Jewish sources for physicians to practise, and indeed for them to be trained and licensed also. This positive attitude, and the close relationship which many Rabbis had with medical matters and the fact that many well known Rabbis of the Talmudic period and later were themselves distinguished physicians could not but have placed in the Jewish mind a positive response to the claims of medicine and its practice. As far as medical training in the Talmudic period is concerned there is little evidence to suggest a formalised programme. Preuss quotes the Midrash (Deuteronomy Rabba 6:13) which mentions a young physician in the company of his master to suggest that training was carried out by the apprentice, attached to the specialist, for a lengthy period of training.[4] This form of medical training was to persist down to the nineteenth century as the mainstay of many a doctor's education.

In normative Rabbinic Judaism, study of the Talmud forms the basis of its main intellectual activity. From this literature emerge the names of many physicians who would act as an inspiration for those in succeding generations. The prime example of Talmudic physicians was Mar Samuel who was born in Nahardea in Babylon in about the year 180. He was a skilled astronomer and some of his legal pronouncements have profoundly affected the Jewish legal system. The Talmud records his pronouncements in many medical areas such as therapeutics, paediatrics, gynaecology and foetal development. However, his medical fame rests on his eye salve which was highly renowned for its effectiveness.

Not all Talmudic references to physicians are complimentary. The taunt that the best of physicians are destined for Gehinnom, a theme also occurring in Greek and Roman literature, has been explained as applying to a physician who harms his patients by not consulting his colleagues because of an exaggerated belief in his own ability.[5] It would also apply to a physician who is haughty or who will not attend to the illnesses of the poor. On balance therefore the traditional Jewish attitude to physicians and the art of healing in medicine is strongly positive. This has influenced many Jews to take up careers in medicine or to combine their medical activities with religious duties as a Rabbi.

During the Middle Ages it was still common for the joint professions of physicians and Rabbis to be held by the same person. It was possible for those learning in Talmudic academies to cover the areas of philosophy and science. Scholars could turn to the practice of medicine to earn their living and indeed many Jewish physicians during the Middle Ages were simultaneously Rabbis, poets and translators, thus possessing a tradition of considerable erudition. Jewish doctors were not only responsible for the care of the Jewish sick but in many cases they attained considerable fame in becoming physician to the leaders of the land in which they were living. The role of the Jewish physician as translator should not be underestimated for Arabic and Greek medical works could be translated into Latin and Hebrew, and vice versa. Thus Jewish physicians helped to transmit Greek medicine to the Arab world and Arab medicine to Europe.

The first Hebrew medical work was composed by Asaph ha-Rofe who lived in the Middle East in the 7th century.[6] The work covers many aspects of medicine and includes a physician's oath. The first medical author in Arabic whose works were brought to Europe was Isaac Israeli (c.855-c.955) who lived in Kairouan in North Africa from the beginning of the ninth century.[7] Previously in Egypt he had been a successful eye doctor and in addition wrote many philosophical treatises on the intellect and the soul. His works on fevers, diet and on urine became standard medical texts which were still in use in the European medical schools many centuries after his death.

It is generally accepted that the first European medical school was founded in Salerno in southern Italy in the ninth century. Traditions abound concerning Jewish involvement in the establishment of this and other early medical schools but no relevant evidence exists. More important was the role of the Jewish physician in Spain from the Arab conquest in the eighth century until the expulsion of the Jews in 1492. This was the period of the 'Golden Age' for the Jews in Spain and they attained high rank at court as well as in every field of scientific, literary and intellectual endeavour. The famous poet Judah Halevi was also a physician as was his contemporary Jonah ibn Bikhlarish (11th century) who compiled a dictionary of drugs in five languages including Greek, Spanish and Latin. The most famous Jewish physician, as well as Rabbi and philosopher, of this period was Moses Maimonides (the Rambam) who was born in Cordoba in 1135.[8] In 1170 he became personal physician to the Sultan of Egypt. Maimonides had a prodigious literary output, including extensive writing on medical matters. He composed an important treatise on asthma, wrote a commentary on the aphorisms of Hippocrates and published *Fusul Musa* ('The Aphorisms of Moses'), which has been translated into many languages. A treatise on hygiene was written in 1197 for the Egyptian Sultan and proved also to be a popular work. Maimonides was a rational physician who disapproved of charms and incantations in treating the sick and who spoke against believing things which were not objectively attested. All this work was carried out against the background of a very busy clinical practice in Cairo. In a letter he sent in 1199 to the colleague and translator, ibn Tibbon, he wrote:

> I dwell at Fostat and the Sultan resides at Cairo; these two places are one and a half miles distant from each other. My duties to the Sultan are very heavy. I am obliged to visit him every morning and when he or any of his children, or any of the inmates of his harem are indisposed I dare not leave Cairo...I do not return to Fostat until the afternoon. Then I am fatigued and hungry. I find the ante-chambers filled with people, both Jews and Gentiles, nobles and common people, judges and bailiffs, friends and foes—a mixed multitude—who await the time of my return.
> I dismount from my animal, wash my hands, and entreat my patients to bear with me while I partake of some food, the only meal I take in the twenty-four hours. Then I go forth to attend to my patients, write prescriptions and directions for their several ailments. Patients go in and out until nightfall and sometimes even, I solemnly assure you, until two hours or more in the night. I converse with and prescribe for them while lying down from sheer fatigue, and when night falls I am so exhausted that I can hardly sleep.

This account of a hectic medical life, allowing rest only on the Sabbath, is at variance with the assertion of Heinrich Graetz that Maimonides was a theoretical rather than a practical physician.[9] Indeed, during this period of intense medical activity Maimonides also served as spiritual leader of Egyptian Jewry, and of Jewries further afield, and managed to produce a continual outpouring of medical, philosophical and legal writing. It was still common during this time for a medical education to lead to positions of power in the Jewish or wider community. However, there is no evidence that Egyptian Jewry, who had much need of his spiritual services, ever objected to the very considerable time input devoted to his medical activities.

Maimonides was content to derive his income from the practice of medicine among Jews and Gentiles.[10] This action was at variance with earlier traditional practice that healing the sick was a religious obligation that should be done without charge, or at most only with re-imbursement for the time lost from other gainful employment. While Maimonides earned his living as a physician he strenuously attacked the growing commercialisation of Rabbinic learning. A greater challenge to scientific medical practice came from the increasing numbers of quacks who utilised charms and incantations and other magic arts on a gullible population. Maimonides himself was a determined opponent of such superstitious activities and his strictures against them had a considerable effect on contemporary Jewish attitudes, although he was never to achieve total success in this area.

The Jewish attitude to the healing art has thus always been strongly supportive and the life of Moses Maimonides who bestrode the two worlds of Jewish learning and medical practice was to be an enduring inspiration to future generations of physicians. While there was little in the practice of their

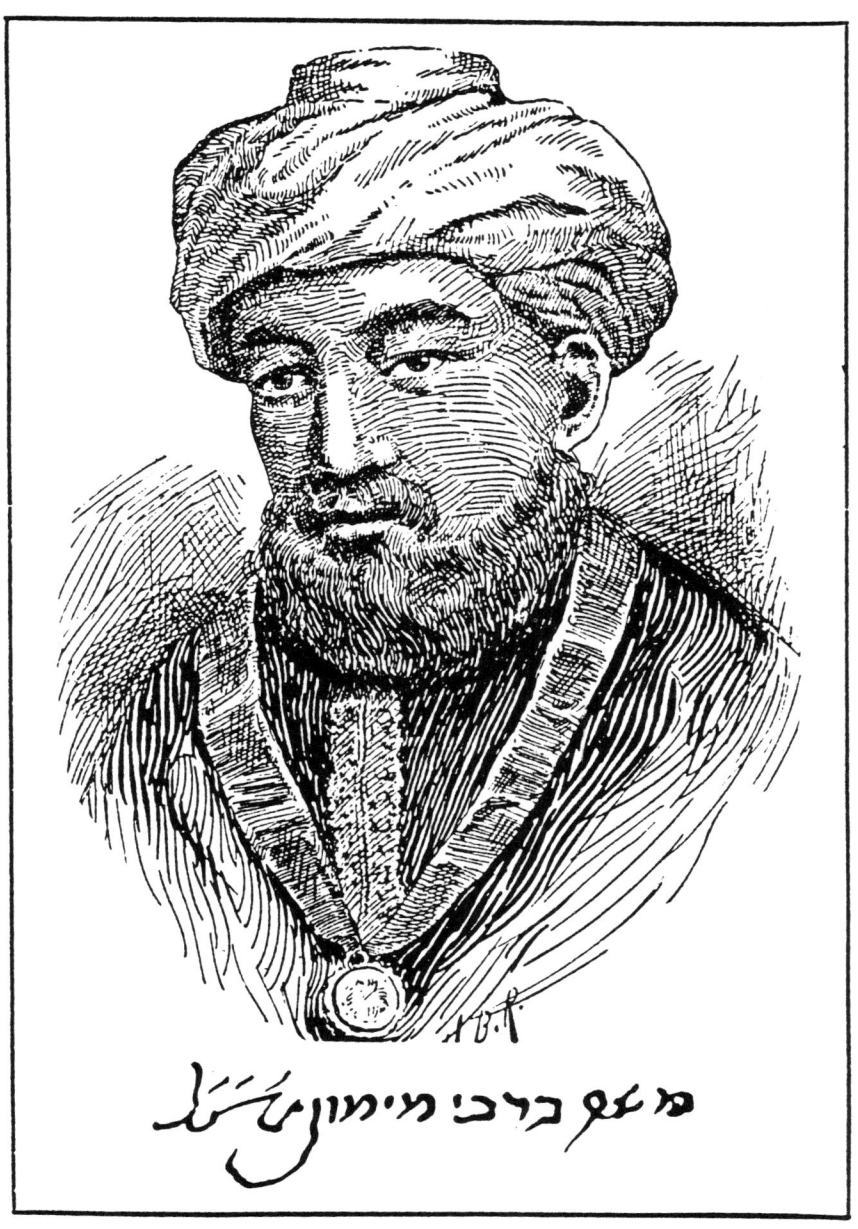

2 Maimonides, philosopher, scholar, Rabbi and physician.

medicine by the mediaeval Jewish physicians which was of a specifically Jewish nature there was no doubt that in the highly segregated life lived by the Jews both in Christian Europe as well as in the Moslem world everything a Jew did was interpreted in terms of benefit or disadvantage to the community.

In the early middle ages an increasing number of Jews were turning to the profession, stimulated by the social advantages offered and secure in the knowledge of religious support for their activities. Salo Baron considers that the number of Jewish physicians at this time must have been large.[11] The cumulative experience of a great many unnamed individuals, transmitted from master to pupil in the course of generations, often enriched medical science far more than did the formal writings which, as Baron notes would less frequently dare to depart from the published works of earlier authorities. The Jewish role in medicine, at the intermediate position between the hostile worlds of Islam and Christendom, was also significant in providing a bridge with the past and offering a sense of continuity in medical developments. The Jewish physician moving with ease between these two worlds would have been able to stimulate the interest of the local population and their practitioners in the new developments taking place in more distant centres.

The era of training physicians by apprenticeship continued in the centuries after Maimonides but the teaching of medicine at the first of the European universities was beginning. Records have been preserved of training contracts between Jewish physicians and their apprentices, and from the prospectuses issued it would appear that schools of higher learning, teaching both Torah and science developed out of these private undertakings.[12] The aim of such institutions was to reduce to a minimum the amount of time required at university to take a degree in medicine. In addition, the student would be exposed to further Jewish studies at a higher intellectual level than would otherwise have been possible. Carmoly has recorded the existence of a Jewish academy in Paris in which medicine was taught and which was said, during the 14th century, to rival the University of Paris.[13]

The high number of Rabbi physicians during the mediaeval period is confirmation that the study of medicine was then regarded as part of a general liberal education. Hippocrates and Galen were the most important authors, but the writings of Israeli and Maimonides were also widely studied. One of the outstanding features of Jewish medicine in this period is the constant emphasis on ethical and social behaviour and the importance of medicine as a service to the community.[14] Medical aphorisms concerning ethical behaviour were composed by every major writer from Asaph to Maimonides although the Physician's Oath long ascribed to Maimonides is today reckoned to have been composed in Germany in 1783 by Marcus Herz, though skillfully composed in the style of Hebrew writing in the twelfth century.[15] While this concern for the ethical and philosophical approach to medicine might have militated against the possiblity of scientific advance the essential contribution of the mediaeval Jewish physicians was their insight into psychological factors in medicine and the importance of mental well-being. The Jewish ritual attention to washing in promoting hygiene and therefore prevention of disease also appears in Hebrew medical writings from the time of Asaph onwards.

From the time of Asaph ha-Rofe there were already a number of small private medical schools in existence. The first European medical school at Salerno has no records of its founding and despite the considerable doubts about the ancient legend that the medical school in Salerno was founded by a Greek, a Latin, an Arab and a Jew each teaching in their own language, there is no doubt that southern Italy in the tenth century did boast a Jewish physician trained in the Greek manner.[16] Shabbetai Donnolo (913-c.982) practised both as a doctor and pharmacist and while no link between him and Salerno has been found his very presence in Italy at this period must have some significance. In addition, Salerno's Jewish quarter had a Jewish physician, Judah, in the year 1005. Donnolo was the first medical writer in Hebrew in Christian Europe and his wide range of medicaments were all derived from the vegetable world. The presence of Donnolo may have given rise to the legend of itself although a notable authority like Baron believes there is a kernel of truth in it.[17]

The earliest universities in Europe were all ecclesiastical establishments and it may be a reflection of the generally unsettled conditions for the small Jewish communities in western and central Europe that no formal action was taken by the Church concerning the attendance of Jewish students at university until the 15th century. Restrictions had been previously placed on the ability of Jewish physicians to practice outside the confines of their own community although such rules were often more observed in the breach.

At the Church Council in Basel (1431-1443) there was a decree, amongst a catalogue of restrictions on Jews, that no Jew should receive a university degree.[18] Regulations were pronounced on Jewish dress, re-affirming the restriction of Jewish residence to the ghettoes and forbidding Jewish physicians to attend gentile patients. It was the university regulations which were new and which emphasised the Christian character of the universities. If Jews attended the colleges they should be made to listen to conversionist lectures and even where special arrangements existed, with Papal authority, at the university in Rome Jews were required to pay additional, and hefty, fees and the oaths required were in Catholic form. Three Jewish physicians and two surgeons were recorded as having taken medical oaths before the Pope in Avignon in the year of 1358 alone.

While the majority of Jewish physicians listed by bibliographers prior to 1800 lived and worked after 1500 this is mainly due to the better survival of records in more modern times; there is ample evidence for earlier extensive Jewish involvement in the medical profession.[19] Indeed there is evidence of Jewish women practising medicine other than the more customary and traditional role in midwifery. There is a notarial record of a Jewish woman doctor in Barcelona in 1388 and many other examples can be found, particularly in Italy and Spain.

One area restricting Jewish medical study was the traditional aversion to dissection of cadavera and this limited surgical practice. It is, therefore, interesting to note the injunction of Isaac Israeli and Moses Maimonides to employ surgery only as a last resort. While Jewish practitioners were acquiring their skills from apprenticeships with older physicians their knowledge of anatomy and surgery would have been limited. This deficiency was corrected only when Jewish students began to attend the university medical schools in the Renaissance era.

Even when Jews found admission to the universities of Europe their problems were far from over. They were subject to special rules and fees. Their graduation fees might be treble those of Christian students and there might be restrictions on their ability to practice. They were, for example, commonly forbidden to treat Christian patients.

Although the award of a medical degree was normally the prerogative of a university education there is some evidence of degrees being awarded without academic authority. There are a number of references of papal grants of licence to practice medicine and orders to examine applicants for medical degrees.[20] These all refer to Jews and have been explained as special dispensation by the Pope in view of the prohibitive decrees of the Church. A remarkable letter patent was sent in 1504 by Pope Julius to Rabbi Samuel Zarfati granting him and his son the right to style themselves doctors of medicine and allowing them to receive all the privileges enjoyed by medical graduates of a university.

After the heyday of Salerno, the University of Montpellier was for a time regarded as the leading medical school. As in Salerno there are legends concerning Jewish involvement in the foundation of the medical school in Montpellier. However, the great Jewish bibliographer Moritz Steinschneider (1816-1907) believed that: 'as in Salerno so in Montpellier, Jews were neither the founders nor the regular teachers.'[21]

Conversely there are university traditions which lend weight to these legends, and contemporary Jewish evidence attests to the number of Jewish physicians then practising in the south of France. A number of these 13th century Jewish physicians were involved in the private teaching of medicine and from the earliest history of the Montpellier school there were a few Jewish physicians, such as Abraham Avigdor in the 14th century who maintained an association with it.

It was the University of Padua, in Italy, which attracted the largest number of Jewish students.[22] The earliest Jewish medical graduate appeared in 1409 and between 1517 and 1721 there were 229 Jews becoming doctors of medicine. A few Jews graduated in Siena up to 1695 and some in Perugia in the middle of the 16th century. It was impossible for Jews to take degrees in Livorno where the medical oath had to be taken on a crucifix. The application of the Canon Law adopted by the Church Council of Basel was still in application in Germany early in the 18th century. An early applicant for admission to the University of Frankfurt (Oder) was Tobias Cohen (1653-1729), the author of the medical work *Maase Tuvia*. The Grand-Elector of Brandenburg over-ruled the Faculty who were unhappy that the Christians, for whom they maintained the university, might be at risk of conversion by being exposed to adherents of the Jewish religion. Cohen and a friend were admitted to study but they were not admitted to examination for degrees and they went to Italy and obtained their degrees in Padua in 1683.

Within the Jewish communities there was increasing opposition to study in universities especially from religious sources fearing for the integrity of Judaism. There were, nevertheless, always traditional Jews who wished to combine contemporary secular knowledge with their sacred studies. In earlier times this could have been carried out within the confines of the Jewish academies of learning, but with the failure to establish a Jewish 'university' in Mantua in 1604, teaching both religious and secular studies, Jews had increasingly to try to enter the general university system.[23]

The movement of Jews into the German universities only took place under the influence of the Enlightenment in the eighteenth century. Jews graduated in Heidelberg from 1728, but there were larger numbers at the University of Frankfurt-am-Oder, nearer the great Jewish communities in Poland, where 130 Jews graduated in medicine in 1810. Polish Jews were attracted to Frankfurt-am-Oder both because of its proximity and because the University of Cracow was closed to Jews.[24] While the University of Halle awarded the M.D. degree to two Jews in 1730 and 1735 it was subject to their promise not to practise in Prussia.

In Poland medicine was the only subject studied by Jews outwith the confines of the Jewish community. This had the result that it was only the Jewish doctor in Poland who possessed secular knowledge at an advanced level within the Jewish community.

Outside Montpellier, the other universities in France, in Paris and elsewhere, were completely under the control of the Catholic Church and they did not admit Jewish students until all the restrictions against Jews were lifted in 1789 with the French Revolution.

Dutch universities began to accept Jews in their departments of medicine from the first half of the 17th century and they were not required to take the Christian oath. During this period the Jewish community in Holland was expanding with an influx of Jewish refugees from the Iberian peninsula where the Inquisition was again becoming active. Jews, who had outwardly been conforming Catholics in Spain and Portugal, were leaving for England, France and Holland as well as the New World. Many were already qualified in medicine and they enriched the medical practice of their new countries.

Once these Iberian emigres, or Marranos, had reached havens of safety they returned in large numbers to the Jewish fold. Most of the first doctors to the poor of the Hebra, the Congregation of Spanish and Portuguese Jews at Bevis Marks in London, were of Marrano origin. Similarly a substantial number of the physicians serving the Jewish community in Poland in the 17th century had a Marrano background. Despite this substantial influx of Jews from Spain and Portugal which continued through the 18th century, though with numbers reducing substantially towards the end of the century, the majority of Jewish physicians in Europe with university qualifications continued to receive their training in Italy and especially at Padua. Indeed, Jews in medicine were generally known as 'Italian doctors' since it was virtually impossible for a practising Jew to become a doctor of medicine outside Italy.

In Spain, nearly all of the great physicians, before the Expulsion of the Jews in 1492, had been Jewish. When outward evidence of Jewish practice had to be concealed the medical traditions continued, in part because of the facilities afforded by medical practice for observance of the Sabbath.[25] Many victims of the Inquisition were Jewish physicians, and the universities, especially the University of Coimbra, had a high proportion of 'New Christian' professors and teachers. Coimbra was, in fact, one of the greatest Marrano centres with almost all the 'New Christians' secret adherents of the Jewish faith. The great Marrano dispersion of the 17th and 18th centuries spread a highly motivated population with a tradition of learning round the Jewish world and to many new areas. The Jews in Jamaica, who supplied many of the first Jewish medical students at the Scottish universities from the end of the 18th century, were substantially of Marrano origin. As Roth observed, the forced assimilation to the general population of a large body of Jews at the close of the Middle Ages allowed the natural talents of the Jews to assert themselves, affording unexampled opportunities for instantaneous advancement.[26] Freed from the previous disabilities there was rapid movement into all areas of intellectual and mercantile endeavour, not merely medicine. It was an example of what might happen in a spirit of freedom of education.

During the seventeenth and eighteenth centuries many thousands of medical students came to Holland to study, especially at the universities of Leiden and Utrecht. Most of the students came from Britain, Scandinavia and from Eastern Europe. Prior to the establishment of the Scottish medical schools, which based their standards on the achievements at Leiden, nonconformist students went abroad for their studies, with a high proportion studying in Holland. It was particularly common to find Scottish and English nonconformist medical students at Leiden at the end of the seventeenth century.

With increasing activity on the part of the Inquisition, especially in Portugal during the seventeenth and eighteenth centuries, large numbers of Marranos settled in Amsterdam. After the northern provinces of the Netherlands proclaimed their independence from Catholic Spain in 1571, after the Treaty of Utrecht, Marranos of Spanish and Portuguese origin were attracted to Amsterdam, where little enquiry was made about their religious beliefs. Synagogues and other religious activities were organised, with the permission of the authorities, from 1614. Jews were thus able to practise their faith openly after more than a century of secret adherence. The magnificent Sephardi synagogue, for Jews of Spanish and Portuguese origin was dedicated in 1675 suggesting a large and settled local Jewish population.

The early practitioners of medicine in the Jewish community in Amsterdam in the seventeenth century were mostly Jewish refugees from Spain and Portugal who were seeking a safe haven in Holland. A few maintained the ancient tradition of combining medicine with religious studies and the Jewish physicians included Rabbis like Aron de Isaac Ledesma, Solomon de Meza, Isaac ben Abraham Uziel and Isaac Naar. Some had been educated in Spain before dropping their Marrano status but from the middle of the seventeenth century Jews were studying in Holland.

The experience of Jewish physicians in Holland suggests that the traditions of combining religious and medical practice continued into the eighteenth century. Of those Jewish physicians listed by G.A. Lindeboom as qualifying before 1780, 43 out of 57 had graduated in the Netherlands while 9 had graduated in Spain or Portugal.[27]

The majority of Jewish practitioners in the Netherlands, certainly until early in the nineteenth century, were in the employ of the Jewish community. They would care for the sick, orphaned or elderly or might have a clientele derived from a wealthier stratum of Jewish society. Thus there were constraints on the levels of Jews in medical practice both because of the limitations in the scope for medical practice as well as the restrictions on Jews entering medical schools.

This pattern of discrimination in the universities of Europe, excluding such exceptions as Leiden, was also to be found in England. As the Jewish community in England increased in size this placed difficulties of intending Jewish medical students. Professing Jews could not take degrees at the Universities of Oxford and Cambridge. At Oxford matriculating students were required to subscribe to the articles of the Church of England. This religious test was required of graduates at the University of Cambridge so that while those unable to subscribe to the articles could matriculate and study at Cambridge they could not receive their degrees there. Jewish teachers at the old English universities, who can be found from the 16th century, were usually converts who had been appointed to teach Hebrew.

The commonly held view that Jews were excluded from Oxford and Cambridge until 1871 when the repeal of the Test Acts swept away the religious tests on both undergraduates and graduates was considerably modified by Cecil Roth.[28] While acknowledging that Jews could not become full members of the universities of Oxford and Cambridge, or be admitted to their fellowships, until the Universities Tests Act of 1871, Roth pointed out the effects of previous enactments on Jews studying there.

Jews who wished to undertake a general university education and were not worried about their inability to graduate could study freely at Cambridge. For example, Natty, Leo and Alfred Rothschild all attended Trinity College, Cambridge to study, though not to graduate, in the period before the lifting of religious restrictions.[29] Alfred Hyman Louis of Birmingham matriculated at Trinity College, and became the first Jewish President of the Cambridge Union in 1850. The first major university reform at Cambridge came in 1856 with the passage of the Cambridge University Reform Act which made it possible for degrees to be taken in Arts, Law, Medicine and Science without religious tests. Membership of the Senate and the holding of university office was, however, still closed.[28]

The Oxford University Reform Act of 1854 opened the lower Bachelor degrees, and matriculation itself, to 'non-declarants' thus creating conditions for Jews to enter and qualify. Thus, while full equality did not come until 1871 there was greater freedom for Jews at the ancient English universities between 1854 and 1871 than is often supposed.[30]

Because of the restrictive policies of the universities of Oxford and Cambridge there was considerable Jewish interest from the outset in the new, secular University College established in London in 1826. Conditions were becoming favourable within Anglo-Jewry during the nineteenth century for an expansion of the university population. In 1815 Anglo-Jewry had been basically a poor community with the majority at susbsistence level or actually on relief. By the eve of the massive wave of immigration from Eastern Europe after 1880 the middle class formed half of the community with the poorer section, while still numerous, now in a minority. The community was developing an English speaking leadership who aspired to a higher education.[31]

By the nineteenth century Jewish acceptance in Britain had been achieved by the successful integration of the community into the mores of the English middle classes. There was pressure on the Anglo-Jewish elite to ensure the rapid integration of immigrant newcomers into the established, and somewhat assimilated, community. Jews were expected to live up to the ideals espoused by the middle classes. Jewish schools and institutions were the means of conferring 'respectability' on the immigrants.[32] Thus, even traditional Jewish characteristics such as the giving of charity, became as much an expression of class interest and social control as were the charitable activities of their non-Jewish neighbours. The priority in the community was anglicisation of the newcomers while the religious immigrant fought valiantly, through newly established chevrot* and benevolent societies, to preserve their independence and culture.

In England, the Jewish community in the middle of the nineteenth century, looked firstly to University College, London for a higher education. Even though some Jews took advantage of the relaxation of the regulations at Oxford and Cambridge from the 1850's the privileges there were not always easily obtained. There had been Jewish links with University College from the outset. It had been founded with the help of one of the foremost emancipationists, Isaac Lyon Goldsmid.[33] Within the Jewish community itself the foundation of Jews College in 1855 was hailed as providing an institution for the Jewish education of the laity. It never achieved this aim and became primarily an institution for the training of ministers in the fashion of other modern Rabbinical seminaries being set up in Western and Central Europe.[34]

In Ireland, the first Jewish graduate was Nathan Lazarus Benmohel, who became Bachelor of Arts in 1836 at Trinity College, Dublin and was therefore the first Jew to graduate in an Anglican university in the British Isles. His graduation was accompanied by the waiver of the Articles of the Church of England. In the years ahead Trinity College had reciprocal arrangements with Oxford and Cambridge for granting degrees *ad eundem* to those with the appropriate credentials.[35]

In Scotland during this period the universities did not require religious tests, which had fallen into disuse a century earlier. Thus the Scottish universities became the mecca for those who were unable, by reasons of conscience, to take up places in the English universities. This was especially so in medicine as the Scottish Universities, alone, allowed Jews to graduate as doctors.

The long standing Jewish obsession with medicine meant that the physician occupied a privileged position in Jewish society, respected by the established

---

* Religious societies.

and assimilated Jews as well as by the more traditional Jewish immigrants. As Anglo-Jewry prospered during the nineteenth century increasing numbers of young Jews aspired to a university education and to a medical training. Unfortunately, the options available for such study were limited in England where the medical degrees at the universities of Oxford and Cambridge were not open to Jews until 1871.

For the Jewish leadership the increasing move into the professions was a vindication of their belief that the Jews could take their true place in society given equality of opportunity. The Anglican establishment were also able to take a benevolent view of Jewish emancipation. It gave Jews the opportunity to advance socially, politically and educationally but the constitutional privileges of the Church of England were maintained and the role of the establishment was left intact.

For Jews seeking to enter medicine or wishing to take some medical studies as an undergraduate, the universities in Scotland offered the best prospects in the eighteenth and nineteenth centuries, until the opening of University College and the rise of the civic universities gave further impetus to the entry of Jews into higher education.

REFERENCES

1. Chaim Bermant, *The Jews* (1977) p.137
2. Julius Preuss, *Biblical and Talmudic Medicine*, trans. Fred Rosner (New York 1977) p.22
3. Immanuel Jakobovits, *Jewish Medical Ethics* (New York, 1967) p.4
4. Julius Preuss op.cit., p.17
5. Fred Rosner, *Medicine in the Bible and Talmud* (New York, 1977) p.152. The Chief Rabbi Immanuel Jakobovits agrees with this explanation viz. *Journal of a Rabbi* (1967) pp. 151-2
6. Fred Rosner op.cit., p.119
7. *Encyclopaedia Judaica* (Jerusalem, 1972) 9, col.1063
8. Harry Freidenwald, *The Jews and Medicine* (Baltimore 1944) 1, pp.193-216
9. Heinrich Graetz, *History of the Jews* (Philadelphia 1891, 1956) 3, p.473
10. Salo Wittmayer Baron, *A Social and Religious History of the Jews*, (New York, 1958) 8, pp. 233-4
11. Salo Wittmayer Baron op.cit., p.255
12. Harry Freidenwald op.cit., p.221
13. E. Carmoly, *Histoire des Juifs Anciens et Modernes* (Brussels 1844) cited in Friedenwald op.cit., p.222
14. Salo Wittmayer Baron op.cit., p.258
15. Fred Rosner op.cit., pp.125-140
16. *Encyclopaedia Judaica* (Jerusalem 1972) 6, cols. 168-9
17. Salo Wittmayer Baron op.cit., p.245
18. Harry Freidenwald op.cit., p.224
19. Salo Wittmayer Baron, *Religious History of the Jews* (New York 1967) 12, p. 84

20 Harry Freidenwald op.cit., pp.263-7
21 ibid., p.241
22 ibid., pp.227, 236
23 ibid., p.221
24 ibid., p.237
25 Cecil Roth, *A History of the Marranos* (Philadelphia 1932) p.177
26 ibid., p.296
27 See G.A. Lindeboom, *Dutch Medical Biography: A Biographical Dictionary of Dutch Physicians & Surgeons 1475-1975*, (Amsterdam 1984)
28 Cecil Roth, 'The Jews in the English Universities', *Miscellanies of the JHSE*, 1V (1942) p.111-2
29 Frederick Morton, *The Rothschilds* (London, 1962) p.165
30 Cecil Roth ibid., p.102
31 V.D. Lipman (ed.) *Three Centuries of Anglo-Jewish History* (1961) p.74
32 Bill Williams, 'The Anti-Semitism of Tolerance: Middle-Class Manchester and the Jews 1870-1900 in A. J. Kidd and K. W. Roberts, eds., *City, Class and Culture: Studies of Cultural Production and Social Policy in Victorian Manchester* (Manchester 1985) pp.77-8
33 Israel Finestein, 'Anglo-Jewish Opinion During the Struggle for Emancipation 1828-1858, *TJHSE* XX (1964) p.126
34 V.D. Lipman op.cit., pp.143-4
35 Louis Hyman, *The Jews in Ireland to 1910* (Shannon 1972) pp.107,142

TWO

Medicine and Education in Scotland

The Scottish universities, especially Edinburgh and Glasgow, have been proud of their international reputation which grew up from the eighteenth century. The international tradition continued into modern times so that substantial numbers of overseas students were attracted to the Scottish medical schools until the outbreak of the Second World War. In 1910 one fifth of all the students at Edinburgh University were from overseas.

This continual attraction of overseas students, which remained a significant theme in Scottish university education, especially in medicine, hinged upon a number of factors. There was an impression that the standard of the medical schools was at the highest international levels and this was combined with ease of entry, religious toleration and economy of fees and living expenses. The overseas students came from the British Empire, the United States of America and Europe, with the relative proportions often depending on local factors in the countries of origin. For Jewish students with a history of exclusion from medical schools in Europe the open access and religious toleration were important. Even the paper qualifications, awarded in absentia in Aberdeen and St. Andrews until the middle of the nineteenth century, had a special significance for Jewish doctors who found these degrees part of their acceptance into British medical society.

As far as the pattern of medical education is concerned, it was during the eighteenth century that decisive changes were made which laid the foundations for important future developments in Scotland. The growth of medical education in Scotland led to the end of the monopoly held by the Universities of Oxford and Cambridge in awarding medical degrees. It also provided a significant challenge to the Royal Colleges by offering an alternative qualification for medical practitioners and by establishing that the university setting was the appropriate one for the provision of medical education. This challenge was later to produce conflict over the opposition of the Faculty (later Royal College) of Physicians and Surgeons of Glasgow to the introduction of the first university degree in surgery at the University of Glasgow in the early 19th century.

The transformation of Edinburgh University from a small college of arts and theology into a major European university with a considerable reputation for medical education was carried out during the early part of the eighteenth century. The Edinburgh Town Council had, uniquely, a controlling interest in the university and they saw in this institution a method of restoring the prestige of their city after the loss of the Scottish Parliament following the Treaty of Union in 1707.

The Edinburgh Town Council were anxious to secure a base for the economic success of their city. They clearly saw that the improvement of the reputation of the university, particularly in the teaching of medicine, would encourage Scottish students to study at home rather than continue to patronise the University of Leiden in Holland. It would also attract high spending medical students from England, Europe and later the colonies.[1,2] The Town Council were the patrons of this development and took an interest in academic appointments. Thus, by the 1750's a well-defined medical professional body was emerging in Edinburgh with the growing confidence that it could direct events. All areas of knowledge were burgeoning during the 'Scottish Enlightenment' and medical progress took place alongside developments in mathematics, natural philosophy, natural history and other subjects.

The reforms which stimulated the improvements in Edinburgh were carried out between 1703 and 1716 while William Carstares was Principal.[3] Carstares instituted changes based on the procedures at Leiden and Utrecht. The systeming of 'regenting', under which students had one teacher for all their studies, was abolished. The students lost some of the close supervision which a good regent could provide, but the new spirit of *lehrfreiheit* enabled professors to become specialists and students to take those courses which interested them most. Carstares' choice of a Dutch model is significant. The Scots had already become used to Dutch medical education, through the numbers of Scots who had studied there from the seventeenth century, and the changes meant that they could have this Dutch-based education more cheaply at home.

It was Carstares' political links with the Monro family which gave further impetus to developments:[3] namely the ideal of creating a medical school in Edinburgh, similar to that in Leiden. The Medical Faculty was founded in Edinburgh in 1726 and over the next thirty years it was to establish, and subsequently maintain, a reputation in international circles for the quality of its medical teaching with a student body recruited from all over Britain as well as from Europe, North America and the West Indies.

The attraction of medical students to Scotland, and particularly to Edinburgh, cannot be solely attributed to the mere fact of the founding of medical schools. There were various factors operating also in those countries from which students were flocking to Edinburgh. Many of the first overseas students came from colonial America. The developing colonies were expanding their populations as new settlers arrived, and it was to be some time before institutions arose which were perceived as being the equivalent of the established medical centres in Europe. Increasing colonial prosperity and developing trade links were additional factors in the close connections between Scotland and North America.[4] It also became common for the sons of emigrant Scots physicians to return to Scotland for their studies, especially after the cessation of hostilities with France in 1748.[5] This continued the Scottish medical tradition into the next generation.

Edinburgh has had a considerable influence on American medicine from the earliest period of colonial history when native Scottish and Scots-Irish physicians established themselves from Massachusetts to South Carolina.[6]

The thistle carved over the door at the medical school of the University of Pennsylvania is a solid tribute to the great Scottish influence on American medicine. The Scottish emigrant physicians helped to form a community of American intellectuals and they continued to maintain links with their alma mater in Edinburgh. They also encouraged young medical students to go to Scotland for their studies.

A number of Americans applied to St. Andrews and Aberdeen for medical degrees, armed with the appropriate letters of recommendation. However, it was Edinburgh's reputation for a comprehensive medical education, and the certificate of competence which its degree implied, which attracted more Americans there than to any other European medical school. Despite this, Edinburgh-trained physicians were still in a minority in America. An apprentice-trained Virginia physician showed his jealousy of those with Edinburgh qualifications when he referred to 'those self swollen sons of pedantic absurdity, fresh and raw from that universal asylum of medical perfection, Edinburgh'.[7]

There was considerable Scottish involvement in the newly founded medical colleges and academies in North America that were being established during the latter part of the eighteenth century. Scots supplied both personnel and the medical curricula which were employed. America had only two medical schools in 1780 but there were 13 in 1820 and this number more than doubled by 1840.[8] The College of Philadelphia had especially close links with Edinburgh as many of its alumni had studied there and both the first provost and first head were Scottish graduates who had been much influenced by their training in Aberdeen and Edinburgh.

A Scottish-style curriculum was also on offer at the College of New Jersey, later known as Princeton University. Benjamin Rush, a signatory of the American Declaration of Independence, studied at the College before proceeding to Edinburgh. The American students in Edinburgh appreciated meeting the leaders of the Scottish enlightenment, like Adam Smith and David Hume. They also enjoyed participating in the social life of Edinburgh which went beyond the taverns and playhouses and included such pastimes as billiards and golf.[9,10] Americans flowed to Scotland and William Cullen, in particular, was reputed to have 'a special measure of esteem for Americans'.[11]

Americans were still attracted to Scotland even after the establishment of the first American medical schools, as subjects in which the Scottish schools excelled, like physiology and anatomy, were not widely taught in America where the rigid classics-based curriculum deterred medical students.[12] Americans were also impressed by the fact that the Scottish universities were benefiting from the enlightenment without severing their ties with the Church.[13] In addition, the Americans, like the Scots, were trying to create a culture that would be both national and cosmopolitan. The conditions were thus being set for a considerable influx of Americans to Edinburgh. By 1800, about 200 Americans had studied medicine in Edinburgh and more than half of them had obtained medical degrees.

In addition the Oxbridge course by its length and its composition did not make itself an attraction to overseas students. In England, medical studies had to be preceded by classical studies, and the full course could take upwards of ten years, mostly in a long and purely theoretical training. Graduation in Scotland did not involve the very lengthy periods of study required by the English universities. In the half century up to 1750, the 617 medical graduates of Oxford and Cambridge exceeded the 406 Scottish medical graduates.[14] In the following half century, the number of Scottish medical graduates increased to over 2,500 while the numbers qualifying from Oxford and Cambridge fell to only 246. The disparity became even more marked in the fifty years up to 1850.

Another major factor in attracting students, including Jewish students, to Scotland was the absence of religious tests. In the seventeenth century many Scots students studied in Holland where medical students enjoyed religious toleration. The proportion of Scots at Leiden was only one third less than the number of English students, and they returned to Scotland determined that the Scottish universities should emulate the medical achievements of Herman Boerhaave (1668-1738) and be open to all who wished to study there.[15] While Oxford and Cambridge were centres of English privilege and ecclesiastical preferment, the Scottish universities saw themselves as part of a broadly conceived national consciousness.

In expanding its student body Scotland accepted students denied access to medical education elsewhere. Catholics, Quakers and Jews came to study in Edinburgh. Religious attitudes were changing in Scotland and the universities were influenced by the liberal and rational ideas then current. These ideas in turn influenced the ministers, who in keeping with Church of Scotland tradition, were university trained. T.C. Smout observed that the appointment of David Hume, Adam Smith, Adam Ferguson and Thomas Reid would have been impossible without some liberty from theological restrictions.[16] In addition, the Church of Scotland was permitted an extra degree of flexibility because many of those who would have opposed changes from within had left to found their own churches during the many episodes of secession between 1740 and 1830.[17]

That the enlightenment took place at all in eighteenth century Scotland implied Church approval endorsing the view of the moderates in the Church that if the Kirk was to have any value in the modern world it must be involved with the new secular developments in the wider world.[18] The growing secularisation meant that the leaders of Scottish society were more concerned with economic growth than their predecessors. At the university it was the study of medicine, rather than divinity, which received most attention. The issues at stake in the universities, including the nature of the new enlightened teaching, were all ultimately settled in favour of the secular interest enhancing the moves towards religious freedoms.[19] This freedom for religion within the university framework does not imply that the second half of the eighteenth century in Scotland was by any means an irreligious age. The Kirk was not seeking to force its own view on every citizen, and through its moderate leadership it lent its own prestige to the achievement of more diffuse Scottish aims, both cultural and economic.[20]

This is not to say that religious tests did not exist in Scotland. They did, and were present in some forms until the middle of the 19th century. For example, the teacher's oath, requiring burgh schoolmasters to subscribe to the Confession of Faith, was removed in 1861 with the passage of the Parochial and Burgh Schoolmasters (Scotland) Act.[21] Within the universities too, there was a modification of the position of religious tests.

James Coutts traces the development of religious tests in the Scottish universities. In the early seventeenth century a religious test was applied so that no student could be enrolled until he had made the confession of faith and religion, as recently prescribed by the Scots Parliament, in the presence of the Principal and regents.[22] The General Assembly of the Church of Scotland in their visitation of 1640, laid down that it should be ascertained 'what conscience each scholler makes of secret devotion, morning and evening'.[23] The Scots Parliament passed an Act in 1662 declaring that the principals, professors and regents in the universities should be 'well affected' to the King and established government. They had to have sanction of the archbishop and take the oath of allegiance in his presence. A few years later, in 1666, philosophy students were also required to take the oath before graduation.[24]

When Presbyterianism was re-established in Scotland in 1690, the Scots Parliament turned its attention to the universities, and on the 4th of July passed an Act which laid down that professors, principals and office-bearers should not be allowed into the universities without taking the oath of allegiance to the Confession of Faith and the Presbyterian form of church government. This was confirmed in the Act of Security which gave a guarantee of permanence to the Scottish universities after the Treaty of Union in 1707.[25] This test was not repealed until 1853 following the election of Lord Dunfermline as Dean of the Medical Faculty of the University of Glasgow in 1841.[26] Lord Dunfermline had declined to take the test, as had been the practice for some time. The dispute which followed took 12 years to resolve.

A petition was presented to Parliament in 1843 pointing out the changes in the Scottish university system since 1707.[26] There were no religious tests before matriculation or graduation and indeed it was felt that such tests would reduce the effectiveness of university teaching. In fact, the Act of Security was not being obeyed. At Edinburgh University, the Chancellor and Rector, as well as the professors, were not being asked to take the oath, except in the Divinity Faculty. It is clear from the accounts that religious tests were not applied to the students; probably they had not been applied from the time of the Act of 1690. In Scotland, religious tests were designed to maintain the religious character of the universities through the maintenance of tests for university office-bearers. However, even these attempts were more often honoured in the breach.[27] At some times and in some places there might be difficulties for those outside the Kirk seeking academic appointments. For students there were no such difficulties. The religious diversity of the student body militated against the introduction of religious tests. There were also powerful economic reasons, in terms of university income, for casting the net for potential undergraduates as widely as possible. Very few Scottish Catholics were attending university in Scotland in the nineteenth century.[28] This does not imply that there was religious discrimination in the universities as the

Catholics' social position excluded them from the traditional channels of mobility. In addition, it was some time before a satisfactory Catholic school network was established in Scotland to provide the local Catholic population with the opportunity to benefit from university entry.[29]

The continuing presence of religious tests at Oxford and Cambridge, even after the reforms of the 1850's, meant that there was always the likelihood that candidates would be attracted to an alternative system. The Scottish universities proved that they were able to attract many who, on geographical grounds, should have been natural entrants to the English universities. In the end the English universities accepted the pragmatic argument that those who were being excluded could study elsewhere, as well as the reformist argument that the tests were inherently unfair.[30]

The cheapness of Scottish university education was also a great attraction. While the young men who set out to be physicians usually came from the upper middle classes, there was also, especially in Edinburgh and Glasgow, a considerable element who came from a poorer stratum in society. Scotland gave students the benefits of a relatively cheap, non-residential university.[31] They met socially in the Edinburgh taverns where the Royal Medical Society meetings were held from the 1740's. The university did not attempt to use residential requirements to impose religious behavioural patterns, such as chapel attendance, on the students. At the end of the eighteenth century the cost of a year's subsistence was only £20 and class fees for a session in the clinical subjects were 3 guineas per subject.[32] The costs for a similar period at Oxford or Cambridge would have been several times higher.

Oliver Goldsmith studied medicine in both Leiden and Edinburgh and he wrote home from Holland that the teaching of 'physic' is much better in Edinburgh and that the expenses in Leiden were much higher.[33] Certainly, it might be expensive for those few students in Edinburgh who lived in the homes of their teachers and professors. Many students in Edinburgh, and the other Scottish universities, in the eighteenth and early nineteenth centuries were extremely frugal, living on sums as small as 6/9 per week.[34] Costs were thus modest by English and international standards and kept open the possibility that many in Scotland with the appropriate talent and the right backing could aspire to a university place.

This attitude, that institutions of higher education should be open to the 'lad o' pairts', was part of the Scottish folk tradition and was an important part of national self-esteem. Although the road might not be easy it was felt that individuals from any background should be able to climb the educational ladder.[35] However, there were few opportunities for social mobility for the urban working class before the changes resulting from the 1872 Education Act.[36] As parochial schools developed in urban centres during the nineteenth century, the social base of medical students widened to include members of the lower middle classes and the new commercial bourgeoisie.[37] Yet even though professional recruitment from the unskilled and those without a priveleged background was limited, it is clear that the Scottish elite in this period was from a wide social range.[38]

The flexibility of the Scottish system was also attractive. Students could study for a period as short as one year and there were no entry requirements. In fact, the open access into the Scottish universities did not end until the introduction of the School Leaving Certificate in 1888. It was only in the medical faculties of the universities that the students followed a prescribed course of study; even there, the heterogeneous student body all had widely varying educational origins.

The students, too, had different educational reasons for visiting Edinburgh for medical study. Some had come from classes in London where there was likely to be a larger supply of material for clinical teaching. Edinburgh had the problem of having a relatively small population with a large student body and there were not always enough patients for clinical teaching. There were also similar difficulties in Glasgow until the opening of the Royal Infirmary in 1794. Many of those who commenced their medical studies in London at the private courses run by William Hunter and George Fordyce were encouraged by these Scottish lecturers to complete their studies in Edinburgh. Others, who were attracted by Edinburgh's reputation, merely wished to spend a year or two there. There were also those who wanted to obtain the medical degree in Edinburgh and many in this group had begun their studies as apprentices to a surgeon or apothecary. A further group of students were graduates of other universities who wished to extend their medical knowledge by seeing for themselves the new medical developments in Edinburgh.

Financial considerations were also important to the teachers. Since the classes were open to all, the professors had an incentive to recruit a large student following which would provide a large income, in the form of fees. Apprentices, intending physicians and even interested lay persons were per-

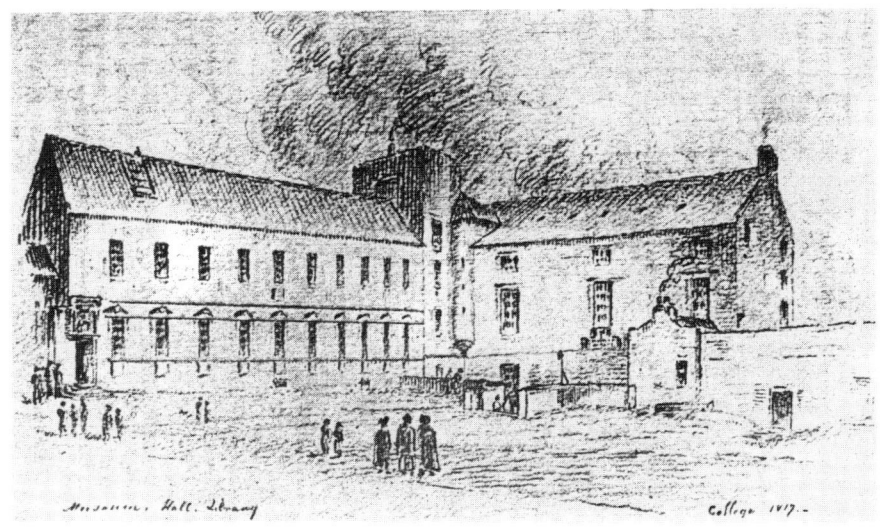

3   University of Edinburgh in the eighteenth century.

mitted to attend lectures and swell class numbers. Students were free to study where they pleased: the awarding of the degree depended on completion of studies but it did not matter where the studies had been conducted. Adam Smith felt that the system of payment by results encouraged the university professors to be sensitive to the needs of their students.[39] Those university classes which were best attended had a high level of enrolment because the teacher was outstanding.

Successful medical teaching guaranteed a good income. By the 1780's the medical professors had become wealthy from teaching, and private practice. Business was so good in Edinburgh that, as the eighteenth century passed, professors passed their own professorial chairs on to their sons. Nepotism reached a peak in the 1790's,[40] but far from this deterring students, the numbers of students attending the anatomy classes, run by the Monros, increased considerably during the eighteenth century from 83 in 1730 to an average of 287 in the decade 1770-1780. After 1800 the numbers increased to over 1800.[41]

The student body benefited from the attention of generations of charismatic lecturers. Joseph Black* appealed to a wide audience and encouraged a large range of Edinburgh folk, such as blacksmiths and druggists, to attend his classes.[42] William Cullen (1710-1790) succeeded, at the relatively late age of 63 years, to the Chair of the Practice of Medicine, where his outstanding reputation as a teacher depended both on his skill as a lecturer as well as his ability to give his students an understanding of the medical theories he was imparting. William Cullen was the first teacher to lecture on medicine in English but there was still considerable emphasis on classical knowledge. This system of education helped to create some of the mystique in the minds of the public about the medical profession. The lecture was the principal teaching method of transferring information from teacher to student to complement the student's own reading.[43] It was popular with the lecturers and cheaper than personal practical experience. Importance was attached to oral teaching, particularly in set lectures. The clinical aspects of the course were also considered important although bedside teaching consisted more of a description of treatment than of any exposition of physical examination and differential diagnosis.[44] However, the Edinburgh Royal Infirmary had a long history of co-operation with the University and it was on the concept of a clinical teaching school that Edinburgh's remarkable success was based.[45]

The commitment to education, which was characteristic of the Edinburgh medical school, was shown in the facilities which grew up in the various attached hospitals and other medical institutions. Andrew Duncan, in particular, who was Professor of the Institutes of Medicine from 1790 to 1819, was active in linking medical education and public health measures. He encouraged the founding of a dispensary in the Old Town and advocated the opening of a mental hospital.[46]

While some students were attracted to Scotland because of religious toler-

---

*Professor of Medicine and Chemistry in Edinburgh from 1766.

ance, economy and the teaching, for many the most important asset of the Scottish universities was their readiness to award the degree of Doctor of Medicine. The degree was seen to be of value in all parts of the medical world, enhancing the career prospects of the holder, except in areas where there were statutory restrictions on medical practice. This was the situation in London where the writ of the Royal College of Physicians ran. There had also been difficulties for surgeons with Scottish qualifications entering the army, navy and East India Company, but these problems were gradually solved between 1788 and 1825.[47] The London colleges did not admit Scottish M.D.s until 1858 but Scottish-trained doctors were free to practise as physicians, surgeons and apothecaries in other parts of England.

With the decline in the use of Latin as the medical lingua franca Scotland attracted increasing numbers of students from other parts of the English speaking world. In addition, the disruptions caused by the Napoleonic Wars deterred many students from attending continental universities.[48] Cullen had been lecturing in English from 1755 although the requirement to present a Latin thesis in Edinburgh was not dropped until 1833. The use of the English language, while helping to sever ties with the continental students, was an important factor in strengthening the links with North America, the West Indies and other parts of the English speaking world. Substantial numbers of Irish Catholics were coming to Scotland to study. Oxford and Cambridge remained in the doldrums in the early nineteenth century and the new English medical schools, based in the new London and provincial teaching hospitals, did not achieve any eminence until the 1820's and 1830's. The Scottish schools held all the advantages for many years.

The Scottish medical influence was enhanced by the dissemination of medical texts, which themselves implied endorsement of the quality of the Scottish medical training. William Cullen's book *First Lines on the Practice of Physick*, completed between 1776 and 1789, was translated into French and German and there were 24 editions printed in such American centres as Boston, Philadelphia and New York, enabling Cullen to exert a powerful influence.[49,50] After the Revolution, the extent of the publishing of Scottish books in America increased enormously.[51]

The unprecedented demand for physicians and surgeons occasioned by the wars in Europe confirmed the centrality of the medical faculty within the universities in Edinburgh and Glasgow. Developments had previously been slow in Glasgow, partially attributed to the lack of clinical teaching material prior to the opening of the Royal Infirmary, and to the conflict between the university and the Faculty of Physicians and Surgeons, who jealously guarded their right, granted under ancient charter, to license practitioners in the greater Glasgow area. However, by the 1820's the Glasgow medical school was beginning to compete seriously with Edinburgh, where the continued reliance on the primacy of lecturing was beginning to sow the seeds of decline by reducing the scope for developing research in the new life sciences.

One of the first signs of local decline in Edinburgh itself was the rapid growth of extra-mural teaching, especially in anatomy.[52] In addition, Edinburgh and Glasgow had to cope with the transformation of medical education in England

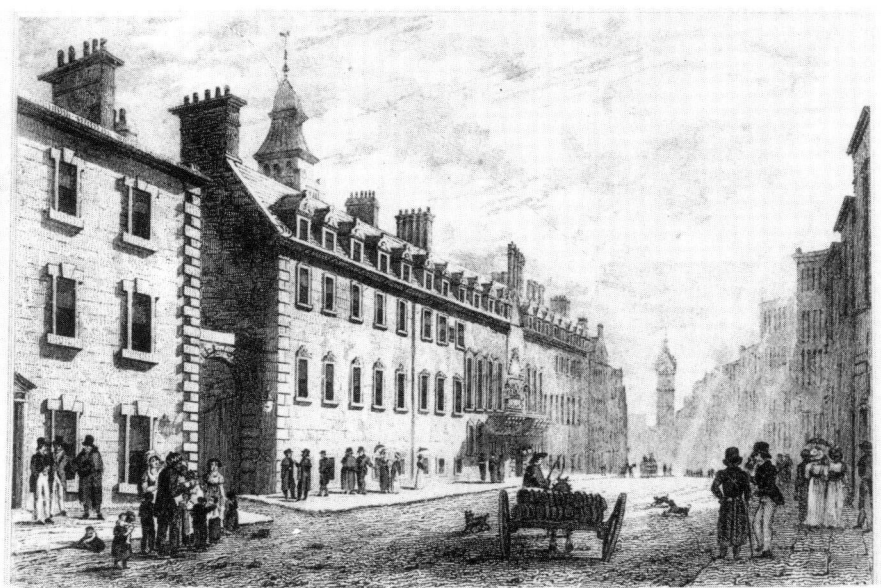

4   University of Glasgow, High Street with the Tolbooth in the distance.

between 1830 and 1858 with the foundation of new medical schools in the large centres of population.

Other factors worked in Edinburgh's favour. With links between Britain and the Continent suspended after 1793 English aristocrats, who would formerly have made the 'Grand Tour', came to Edinburgh. The city was a pleasant place to live and work in and the commercial success of the Edinburgh publishers and booksellers meant that the city's thinkers and writers could receive substantial advances for their works.[53]

The medical degree proved to be an attraction in itself. While some surgeons declined to take this optional degree, usually because of the expense, it became customary for many to request the degree later in life. The degree remained popular even if it was possible to practise without it. The ideal of crowning the undergraduate career with the medical degree led to the growth of professional coaches, or 'grinders', who would, for a fee, provide various services for the students.[54,55] Students would be coached in examination technique, important for a Latin oral, and might be taught the Latin stock phrases which might impress an examiner. Some grinders even had a stock of Latin theses, or at least would considerably edit the original works of students, to better guarantee success.

While the reputations of the medical schools in Edinburgh and Glasgow were increasing, it remained the practice at Marischal College and King's College in Aberdeen, and in St. Andrews for the M.D. degree to be awarded *in absentia*. While efforts were made to ensure that the applications were in order, and were supported by affidavits by at least two established practitioners, the practice was open to abuse. In Edinburgh and Glasgow, this form of degree awarding was stopped in the middle of the eighteenth century and regulations were further enforced at the beginning of the nineteenth century. These stipulated the required period of study and which subjects were compulsory. The ability to study in one university and graduate at another was not affected.

It was simpler to graduate *in absentia* from Aberdeen or St. Andrews. The University of St. Andrews had possessed the right since 1414 to award medical degrees. It had occasionally taught the subject but from 1696 it had been selling doctorates without providing any medical teaching.[56] In 1722 Thomas Simson was appointed to the chair endowed by the Duke of Chandos but the position of the chair was unsatisfactory from the start. Very soon its function was to confer medical doctorates in ever increasing numbers. All that might be said in St. Andrews' defence was that other universities also had liberal attitudes and the substantial income from this trade may even have saved the university from bankruptcy during the eighteenth century.[57] In 1799, provision was made for an examination in St. Andrews but until 1826 the degree could still be awarded *in absentia*. After this date proof of training and passing a final examination was required but the St. Andrews degree still attracted a large number of practitioners. In 1845 no fewer than 106 obtained the M.D. in this way, at a cost of 25 guineas each, of which the government received £10 for stamping the medical diploma.[58]

Aberdeen which had a mediciner from 1494 possessed two degree-awarding institutions, Marischal and King's Colleges, until 1860. The small size of these colleges and their constant bickering prevented the development of a significant medical school. In addition, their readiness to award medical degrees, on the basis of affidavits, enabled those ill-disposed to Scottish medicine to attempt to cast suspicion on all Scottish degrees.

Besides the financial advantage accruing to Aberdeen, the system enabled many experienced practitioners to gain additional respect, or to charge higher fees. As long as the system was policed properly those being awarded degrees on the basis of affidavits could be as worthy doctors as those completing studies in Edinburgh under the tutelage of the grinders.

Adam Smith defended the practice because he felt that the desire by certain practitioners for the style of doctors was harmless, and would not fool anyone.[59] In any case Smith did not want to see a monopoly developing in the awarding of medical qualifications. Doubts remained about the degrees until reforms were instituted. There was a sharp drop in the number of graduates in Aberdeen after the rules were tightened there in 1825 but St. Andrews continued in its own way until the passing of the Medical Act in 1858. The popularity of the Scottish degree, among medical practitioners, was never in any doubt. They remained much sought after in all the Scottish universities and between 1750 and 1850 over 90% of all British medical graduates received their degrees from the Scottish universities.*

---

*See table 5:1, D. Hamilton, *The Healers* (Edinburgh 1982) p.151.

The prodigious output of medical graduates helped to produce the leaders of medicine in Britain and abroad in the nineteenth century.[60] Many of the new English medical schools, such as those in Liverpool and Manchester, as well as Barts and the Middlesex in London, were founded by Scottish graduates. The Dublin medical school owed its origins to such Edinburgh graduates as Cheyne, Stokes and Corrigan. Canadian medicine was greatly influenced by Scotland; the Medical Faculty at McGill University grew out of a private medical school founded by a group of doctors who had trained in Edinburgh.

In Russia too, Scots physicians were to be found,[61] involved in all aspects of medical practice. The Indian Medical Service owes an especial debt to the work of Scots physicians as fully half of the Indian Medical Service, from the seventeenth to the twentieth century, was Scottish,* indicating that the prodigious output of the Scottish Medical schools had to find employment prospects in colonial and army service. Links between Scotland and Australia go back to 1883 when Thomas Anderson Stuart, an Edinburgh graduate, began the Sydney medical school.[62] The connection with Dunedin, in New Zealand, was especially close as the town was planned by the New Edinburgh Settlement. Edinburgh graduates were involved with the start of the Otago Medical School and the links thus forged remained strong. In the United States, as we have seen, the Edinburgh medical input had been strong from the start of the provision of medical education and medical services there. Edinburgh flourished on the success of its graduates all over the world.

Despite their shortcomings, the Scottish universities continued to be able to provide an educational system which developed the traditional Scottish machinery designed to neutralise the inequalities of scholastic and family background.[63] There were no religious bars to progress and the way was always open for anyone with the determination and ability to succeed in achieving their ambitions. The quality was high, entry was open and it could hardly have been cheaper.[64]

This preponderance of medical graduation in Scotland decreased after 1850: one of the many changes taking place in British medical training. These changes were taking place against the background of a British debate about the role of education and science. The expanding middle class demanded a widening of the university curriculum and new subjects either began to be studied after 1870 or received a greater emphasis. The Victorian period saw the growth of the English civic universities of which the new provincial medical schools formed part. Medicine was now becoming a graduate profession and though medical training by apprenticeship had still been commonplace in Edinburgh in 1830 it had become obsolete twenty years later.[65] These changes were also occurring in England; in 1827 fewer than 6 out of 6000 members of the Royal College of Surgeons had been university graduates.[66]

Changes were also occurring within the Scottish school system which affected university entrance. Students were older, with few now entering below the age of fifteen. The old parochial school network was unable to cope with comprehensive coverage of the whole population, and the failure of

---

*See D. G. Crawford, *Roll of the Indian Medical Service 1616-1930* (1930).

adequate state support for the secondary schools meant that those emerging from these schools were unable to achieve their full potential. The secondary schools became the main feeder for the university system with the parochial schools diminishing in importance although in the Highlands and North East of Scotland local developments in the parochial school network produced a significant number of working class university students.[67]

However the general ethos of Scottish education had not changed. It sought to provide the bulk of the population an elementary education while offering a smaller number of children the opportunity of a higher education which would qualify them for an elite rôle in society.[68] Scottish entrants into the professional elites thus did not necessarily come from any families further down the social scale than their English colleagues and Scottish privilege might stand in the way of the 'lad of pairts'.[69] The opportunity to study at a Scottish university was several times greater for the sons of ministers, doctors and teachers and, to a lesser extent, farmers, than for the sons of shepherds, miners or blacksmiths.[70] The sons of artisans did not enter university from school but after some years at work. Nevertheless the claim that the universities were promoting social mobility is still valid when it is remembered that only about half of the students' fathers had studied at university themselves. Scotland had one university place for every 1,000 of the population in the 1860's, a level almost six times that of England.[71] The survival of the parochial school led to the perpetuation of the 'democratic myth' in Scottish education, that all could obtain such an education as would enable them to reach that position in life for which their talents and character would allow. The possibility of improvement did exist and was open but the way was not too easy, as ambition, hard work and moral resolution, as well as talent, were required.

Economically, Britain was experiencing a boom during the 1870's but with the economy later slowing down, and the fear of German technological expansion, there was an upsurge in scientific and technical education. In Scotland this produced considerable expansion in the existing universities and the formation of a new university college in Dundee, the first in Scotland since the Middle Ages.[72] In this expansion the medical schools were especially successful in their levels of recruitment.[73] The average age of the students was beginning to rise but the social composition of the students remained unchanged. Thus, the universities were giving a semblance of truth to the democratic myth.[74] In the early 1860's the Scottish Arts Faculties took 23% of their intake from children of manual workers, many as young as 13 or 14 years old, straight from parochial school. There was a penalty to pay for this open door. The universities became regarded as alternatives to the burgh schools, often catering for the same students and not making much higher demands, though this did not apply, obviously, in the vocationally orientated medical faculties.

The introduction of the Higher Leaving Certificate, in 1888, meant that more rigorous entry standards to universities were being employed. However, recruitment to the Scottish universities at the end of the Victorian period continued to encompass a wide section of society. Thus, talented individuals could be selected for social promotion at the expense of those whose resources, whether intellectual or financial, rendered them incapable of making any educational advancement.

The Scottish universities grew in size as the academic standards improved. From 4,400 places in 1830 they advanced to 6,000 in 1900 increasing to 10,000 in 1938.[75] With the founding of the Carnegie Trust for the Universities of Scotland there was an improvement in the level of availability of bursaries. By 1910 the Carnegie Trust helped with the fees of about half of the university students in Scotland. At Glasgow, the percentage of working-class students reached 24% in 1910, a level which remained unchanged over the next fifty years.[76] The characteristic ambition of a child of Scottish working-class parents entering university in the first decades of the twentieth century was to aim to be a teacher. A child from Social Class 1 was 80 times more likely to enter medicine than one from Social Class V.

The nineteenth century also saw the development of extra-mural medical schools, so called as they grew up outside the universities.[77] The oldest was the Anderson's College Medical School in Glasgow which was opened in 1796 as part of a greater plan, which was not realised, for a new university. Extra-mural teaching in Edinburgh dated back to the eighteenth century and during the nineteenth century distinct schools were formed. However, it was not until 1895 that the Medical School of the Royal Colleges of Edinburgh was formally set up.[78] St. Mungo's College was founded as the medical school of the Glasgow Royal Infirmary in 1876 after teaching facilities had been transferred to the Western Infirmary following the removal of the University

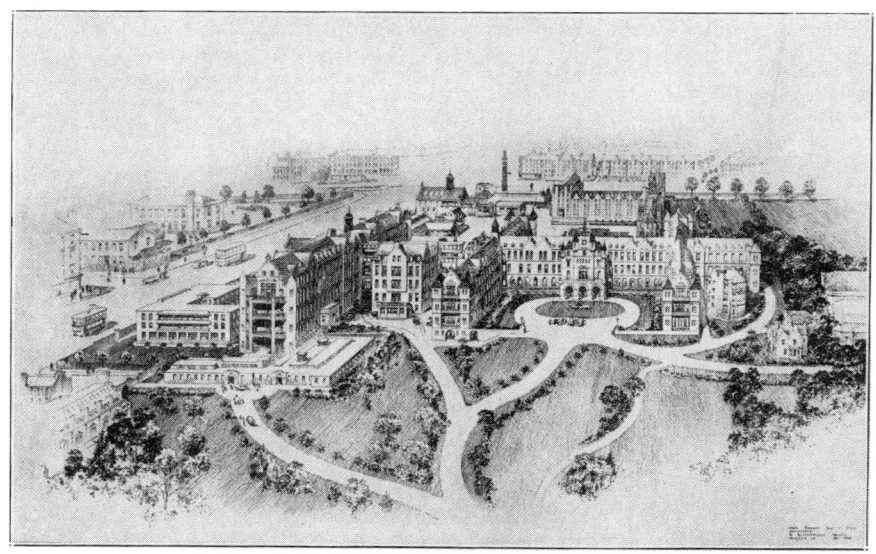

5   Western Infirmary, Glasgow, 1874.

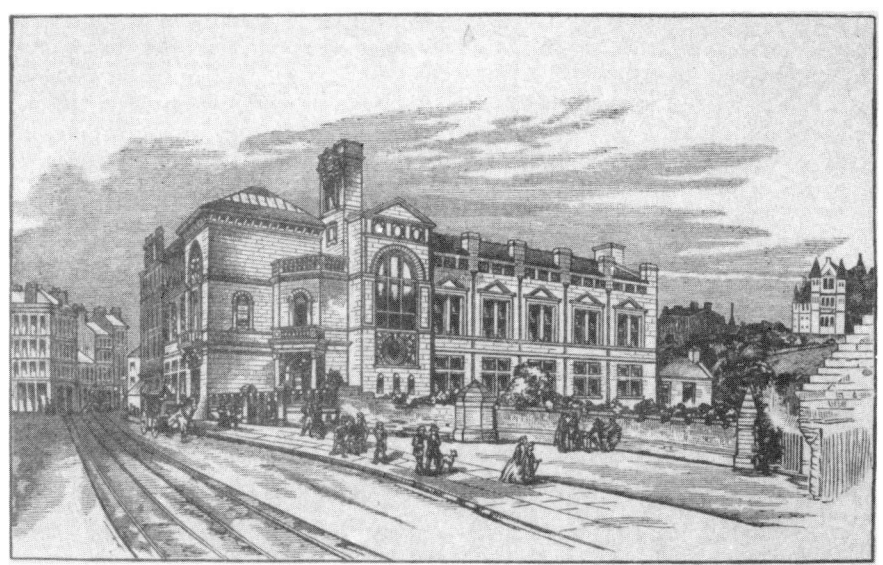

6 Anderson's College of Medicine, Glasgow.

of Glasgow to Gilmorehill.[79] Extra-mural teaching had reached a peak of success in Glasgow and Edinburgh between 1840 and 1860 but the number of students later declined and it was only the arrival of overseas students in the twentieth century which guaranteed their survival into the 1940's.

By the twentieth century the basic philosophy in Scottish education was to make available public secondary education to those whom they felt could benefit by it, and to make it appropriate for the future career needs of the pupils. Children were streamed into academic and non-academic groups by the age of twelve, with the former group mainly, but not entirely, middle class and the latter group working class. The 'lad o' pairts' aspect of the democratic myth became transformed into opportunity based on ability which satisfied the contemporary ideals of equal opportunities.[80] A small number of gifted poorer children might make it to the top, if given an unusual degree of support by parents and teachers, even if most were to remain in the social class of their birth.[81] Scottish education was meritocratic rather than democratic giving support to those able to climb the social ladder.[82]

Thus, the conditions in the Scottish universities made it possible for the growing Jewish community in Scotland to direct its sons into higher education, and especially into medicine. The system was open to those who had the financial resources to meet the fees and the determination to pursue an undergraduate career. Financial sacrifice by eager parents was topped up by assistance from Carnegie grants. As the children of the wave of East European Jewish immigrants, who entered Scotland between 1880 and the outbreak of the First World War, completed their schooling in Scotland the conditions were set for an ever increasing proportion of Jewish students in the Scottish universities. This concentration was most obvious in Glasgow where the bulk of Scottish Jewry was to be found in the twentieth century, proving that it was possible for a group of students, of humble origins, to enter the Scottish universities given their unusual determination to succeed.

REFERENCES

1. Anand C. Chitnis, *The Scottish Enlightenment* (1986) p.138
2. Stephen Shapin, 'The Audience for Scottish Science', *Hist. Sci* xii, (1974) p.97
3. ibid., p.84
4. Helen Brock, 'Scotland and American Medicine', in William Brock, *Scotus Americanus*, (Edinburgh 1982) pp.114, 118
5. ibid., p.117
6. John Z. Bowers, 'The Influence of Edinburgh on American Medicine', in Gordon MacLachlan, (ed.) *Medical Education and Medical Care: A Scottish-American Symposium* (1977) p.4
7. William G. Rothstein, *American Physicians in the Nineteenth Century*, (Baltimore 1972) p.36
8. ibid., p.93
9. Helen Brock op.cit., p.122
10. D.B. Horn, *A Short History of the University of Edinburgh 1556-1889* (Edinburgh, 1967) p.91
11. Andrew Hook, *Scotland and America* (Glasgow 1975) p.23
12. John Z. Bowers op.cit., pp.6-7
13. ibid., p.8
14. A.H.T. Smith, 'Medical Education at Oxford and Cambridge prior to 1850' in F.N.L. Poynter, *The Evolution of Medical Education in Britain* (1966) p.49
15. E. Ashworth Underwood, *Boerhaave's Men at Leyden and After*, (Edinburgh 1977) pp.4,24
16. T.C. Smout, *A History of the Scottish People 1560-1830*, (1969) p.232
17. ibid., pp.233-7
18. Anand C. Chitnis op.cit., pp. 52-3
19. ibid., p.158
20. T.C. Smout op.cit., pp.236, 239
21. Ian R. Findlay, *Education in Scotland* (Newton Abbot 1973) p.19
22. James Coutts, *A History of the University of Glasgow* (Glasgow 1909) p.57
23. ibid., p.107
24. ibid., pp.147-8
25. ibid., pp.165-89
26. ibid., pp.419-21
27. Anand C. Chitnis op.cit., p.157
28. R. D. Anderson, *Education and Opportunity in Victorian Scotland : Schools and Universities* (Oxford 1983) p.305
29. Sister Martha Skinnider, 'Catholic Elementary Education in Glasgow: 1818-1919' in T.R. Bone (ed.) *Scottish Education: 1872-1939* (1967) p.14

30 Charles Newman, *The Evolution of Medical Education in the Nineteenth Century* (1957) p.277
31 J. B. Morrell, 'Medicine and Science in the Eighteenth Century', in Gordon Donaldson (ed.) *Four Centuries: Edinburgh University Life* (Edinburgh 1983) p.43
32 David Hamilton *The Healers* (Edinburgh 1982) p.121
33 J. D. Comrie *History of Scottish Medicine* 1, (1932) p.339
34 ibid., p.350
35 R. D. Anderson, op.cit., p.2
36 ibid., p.336
37 ibid., p.319
38 ibid., p.339
39 David Hamilton ibid., p.120
40 J. B. Morrell op.cit., p.40
41 J. D. Comrie ibid., p.320
42 J. B. Morrell op.cit., p.48
43 Charles Newman op.cit., p.26
44 ibid., p.26
45 Anand C. Chitnis op.cit., pp.183-4
46 ibid., p.183
47 David Hamilton op.cit., pp.139-45
48 Ella Hill Burton Rodger, *Aberdeen Doctors at Home and Abroad* (Edinburgh 1893) p.167
49 Ralph H. Major, *A History of Medicine* (Oxford 1954) p.590
50 John Z. Bowers op.cit., p.20
51 Andrew Hook op.cit., p.78
52 D. B. Horn op.cit., p.109
53 Anand C. Chitnis op.cit., p.38
54 D. B. Horn op.cit., p.106
55 J. D. Comrie op.cit. Vol. 11, p.478
56 Douglas Young, *St. Andrews* (1969) p.204
57 R. G. Cant, *The University of St. Andrews* Edinburgh 1946), pp.86, 100
58 ibid., p.247
59 James Coutts ibid., pp.508-10
60 Ronald Girdwood, 'Edinburgh in the History of Medicine' in Gordon MacLachlan (ed.) *Medical Education and Medical Care: A Scottish-American Symposium* (1977) pp.34-42
61 W. Horsley Grant, *Russian Medicine* (New York 1937), pp.68,70
62 W.S. Craig, *History of the Royal College of Physicians of Edinburgh* (Oxford 1976) p.376
63 George E. Davie, *The Democratic Intellect: Scotland and her Universities in the Nineteenth Century* (Edinburgh 1964) p.xxvii
64 W.M. Mathew, 'The Origins and Occupations of Glasgow Students: 1740-1839, *Past and Present* XXX111 (1966) pp.92-3
65 J. D. Comrie op.cit. Vol. 11, p.340
66 Michael Sanderson (ed.), *The Universities in the Nineteenth Century* (1975) p.60
67 R. D. Anderson op.cit., p.182
68 T. C. Smout, *A Century of the Scottish People* (1986) p.218
69 Robert Anderson, 'Secondary Schools and Scottish Society', *Past and Present* (1985) p.209
70 R. D. Anderson op.cit., p.152
71 T. C. Smout op.cit., p.216
72 Michael Sanderson op.cit., p.145

73　R. D. Anderson op.cit., p.294
74　T. C. Smout op.cit.
75　David Hamilton, *The Healers*, (Edinburgh 1982) p.150
78　W. S. Craig, *History of the Royal College of Physicians of Edinburgh* (Oxford 1976) p.342
79　*Glasgow Royal Infirmary Report for 1947*, in Greater Glasgow Health Board Archives, p.6
80　ibid., p.340
81　T. C. Smout op.cit., p.225
82　Robert Anderson, 'Education and Society in Modern Scotland—A Comparative Perspective', *History of Education Quarterly* 25 (1985) p.478

THREE

Jews in Medicine in Scotland Before 1880 and the Development of the Immigrant Tradition

The entry of Jews into medicine in Britain followed the arrival of Jews in Britain from the Iberian Peninsula and Central Europe. Unable to achieve medical education or qualifications from the English universities some turned to Scotland to further their ambitions. Only small numbers of Jews qualified in medicine in Scotland in the two hundred years between the re-establishment of the community in London in 1656 and the eve of the great Jewish immigration to Britain from 1880. Nevertheless these figures must be seen against the small size of the Anglo-Jewish community and its precarious status as a predominantly immigrant group.

The first Jews to enter medicine not only established a trend within the community but they reasserted the Jewish interest in medicine so that the Jewish physicians in Britain formed part of the long chain of Jewish medical tradition. In Scotland this was epitomised by the career of Asher Asher who was born to poor Polish immigrants in Glasgow and, as will be seen, became a successful doctor, firstly in Glasgow and then in London. Asher's career still forms part of Glasgow Jewry's folk legacy and was a powerful stimulus to his later co-religionists who wished to follow the same path.

As previously discussed, Jews began to settle in Britain after the resettlement in 1656. At first most Jews arrived in Britain via Amsterdam where a substantial Marrano population had grown up. In addition to those Jews who arrived through Amsterdam there was a steady influx of Jews directly from Spain and Portugal during the eighteenth century, though with diminishing numbers as the century progressed

From the earliest period of the Jewish community in London it became the practice of the Synagogue of Spanish and Portuguese Jews to appoint a physician to serve the Jewish poor. As the numbers of Jews increased during the first half of the eighteenth century it became necessary to appoint a second doctor. It had become established that the Hebra, as the Spanish and Portuguese community was called, required both a surgeon and a physician and there were even occasions when the pressure of work in the poor, sick immigrant population demanded the attention of a third physician.[1]

Initially, Jewish doctors serving the Hebra had received their training in Portugal prior to their settling in Britain. Lack of a medical qualification was not a bar to medical practice in the eighteenth or early nineteenth centuries. It was possible to practise outside London or to confine activities exclusively within the Jewish community. In the London 'sister' congregation in Amsterdam the majority of the Jewish practitioners were employed in the various

Jewish philanthropic organisations or supplied the medical needs of others within the Jewish community. Many of the first Jewish physicians in London were content to work without a British qualification but gradually there was an interest in obtaining a British degree. Even so, employment by the Hebra remained a valuable career option for Jewish practitioners well into the nineteenth century. With Oxford and Cambridge closed to professing Jews, the only avenue for a university degree was in Scotland.

There were almost no Jews resident in Scotland in the eighteenth century and communities were not officially established until the first decades of the nineteenth century. Therefore, Jewish students who came to study in Scotland, almost exclusively in Edinburgh, were attracted by the medical opportunities available yet lacked the support of local Jewish families to bid them welcome.

The first Jewish medical students in Scotland date from 1767 in Edinburgh but Jews had been graduating in medicine in Aberdeen for almost thirty years before that. From the records of Marischal College and King's College, in Aberdeen, the names of sixteen Jewish medical graduates between 1739 and 1824 can be identified. (Table 3:2–see p.37) With only two exceptions all these practitioners were based in England, primarily in London. It is likely that the obtaining of such a medical qualification would have had some value in promoting career advancement as well as enhancing the prestige, and thus fee charging ability of the holder. For the Jewish community, mostly composed of new immigrants from Iberia and Central Europe, the degree was an indication of acceptance into the mainstream of British medicine.

The first Jew to graduate in Aberdeen was Jacob de Castro Sarmento (1691-1762) who received his M.D. in July, 1739.[2]* The contemporary records of Marischal College have not survived but the awarding of a medical degree to such a prominent member of the Jewish community must have represented something of a test case. In addition, the doctors supplying the affidavits for Sarmento's degree included Sir Hans Sloane, then President of the Royal Society, thus conferring additional respectability on the qualification obtained.

Sarmento was, for a time, involved in the medical service of the Hebra and was involved in the foundation of the Bet Holim, the first hospital of the Jewish community in London. In the following years there were numerous physicians and surgeons who served the community and were appointed to serve the Bet Holim. The doctors working for the Hebra in the eighteenth century were mainly of Iberian origins and most were content to work without a local medical qualification but as time went on more followed Sarmento's path and took degrees in Aberdeen (Table 3:1).

The acquisition of a medical degree was, therefore, useful to a medical practitioner since it was obtained later in a professional career. In addition to enhancing prestige it served to provide the stamp of British legitimacy to

---

*For biographical details of Sarmento and other Jewish medical students and graduates in Scotland before 1880 see Appendix 1.

Table 3:1 Doctors of the Hebra who studied or graduated in medicine in Scotland

	Date of graduation or of studies
Jacob de Castro Sarmento	1739
Joseph Hart Myers	1779
Solomon de Leon	1786-88
Benjamin Lara	1802
Emanuel de Asher Pacifico	1817
Judah Israel Montefiore	1824

foreign practitioners who wished to settle in Britain. For the Jewish refugees from the Inquisition in Portugal, the Aberdeen diploma was the best source of obtaining a British medical qualification. Oxford and Cambridge were closed to them and they would have had no desire to engage in further studies by taking classes in Edinburgh or Glasgow.

The authorities in Aberdeen looked on the medical degree as a legitimate reward for medical services carried out by experienced practitioners who had been recommended for the honour by their medical peers. Others looked on the awards more cynically, regarding them as a means of obtaining revenue for the college. However, the Aberdeen colleges did not make a lot of money out of awarding degrees *in absentia* as only about half a dozen awards were made each year. Jacob de Castro Sarmento's M.D. degree was only the 14th awarded by Marischal College and six years later, Ralph Schomberg became the College's 29th medical graduate.[3] They also attempted to ensure that the holders of their diploma were worthy of the honour, although, as will be seen, they were not always successful in this as the following eighteenth century jingle confirms:[4]

> Ne'er doubt my pretensions I am a physician
> See here's my diploma and in good condition,
> From Aberdeen sent by the coach on my honour,
> I paid English gold to the generous donor.

Nevertheless, the process of graduating *in absentia* had the benefit of enabling a number of distinguished Jewish practitioners to obtain medical qualifications which would have otherwise been unavailable to them.(Table 3:2) Sarmento, Lewisohn, Lara and many others pursued worthy medical careers in Britain and abroad and the precedent thus established continued well into the twentieth century with a few Jews amongst the large number of medical practitioners graduating in Aberdeen and St. Andrews without having studied there first.

While many of the graduates were highly regarded in their professional life, only Nathaniel Wallich (1786-1854) has an entry in the *Dictionary of*

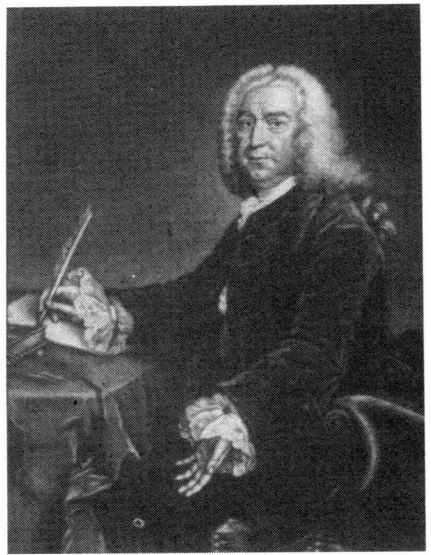
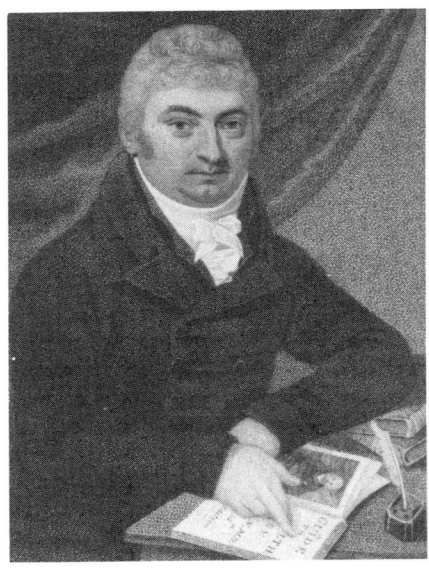

7 Jacob de Castro Sarmento graduated at Marischal College, Aberdeen in 1739.

8 Samuel Solomon who made a fortune from the sale of the Cordial Balm of Gilead.

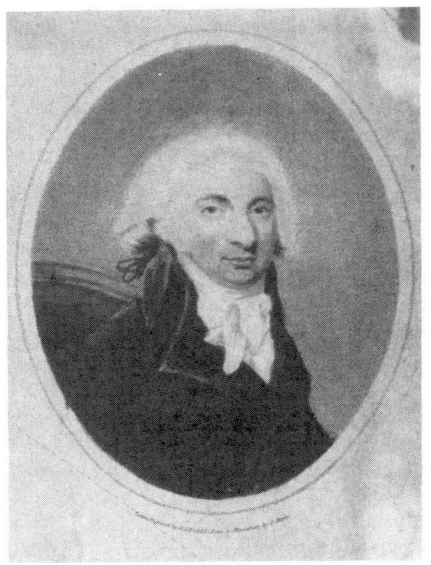
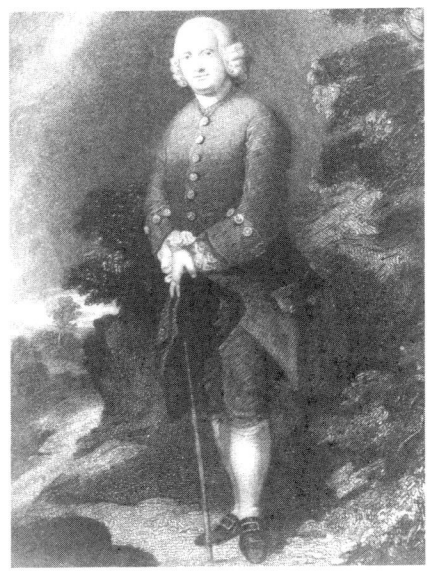

9 William Brodum, author of 'A Guide to Old Age', whom Marischal College sought to 'de-graduate'.

10 Ralph Schomberg, physician and plagiarist.

Table 3:2 Jewish Medical Graduates in Aberdeen before 1880

(a)
Marischal College

Year	Name	attested by
1739	Jacob de Castro Sarmento	Sir Hans Sloane, Dr. Alexander Stewart, Dr. Cromwell Mortimer.
1745	Ralph Schomberg	Dr. J. Colex, Dr. Leon Welsted, Dr. M. Schomberg, Dr. John Phillipson.
1755	David Cohen	good attestations from London and Edinburgh.
1775	Gumpertz Lewisohn	Dr. Smith, Dr. Wilson.
1783	Benjamin Lyon	
1791	William Brodum	Dr. Saunders, Dr. Luis Leo.
1796	Samuel Solomon	Dr. Joseph Moore, Dr. Isaac Fisher.
1802	Benjamin Lara	Dr. Jamieson, Dr. Thomson
1814	Joseph da Cunha	Dr. George Pearson, Dr. Richard Harrison, Dr. P.M. Roget.
1816	Jacob Adolphus	Sir James M'Gregor, Dr. Edmond Sommers
1819	Nathaniel Wallich	Dr. Hamilton, Dr. Fleming.

source: Officers and Graduates of University and King's College, Aberdeen 1495-1860, 11, (ed.) P.J. Anderson, (Aberdeen 1893)

(b)
King's College

Year	Name	attested by
1816	Daniel Baruh	Dr. J. Sequira, Dr. Joseph Hart Myers
1817	Emmanuel Pacifico	Dr. Sutherland, Dr.Babbington Dr. Joseph Hart Myers.
1824	Judah Israel Montefiore	Dr. Algernon Frampton, Dr. John Meyer.
	Daniel Garcia	Dr. John Meyer, Dr. John Ramsbotham.
1859	Samuel Cardozo	

source: Officers and Graduates etc.

National Biography on account of his contribution to Indian flora.[5] Wallich was awarded an M.D. by Marischal College in Aberdeen in 1819, and this must have been a useful qualification to a foreign graduate.

His son, George Wallich came to Edinburgh University in 1832, graduating M.D. in 1836 with a thesis 'on pneumonia', and followed his father into service in the Indian Medical Service. Thus while Nathaniel Wallich was a Scottish medical graduate *in absentia* his son had a regular undergraduate career in Edinburgh. This progression from graduation *in absentia* to formal undergraduate study in Edinburgh was also followed by Abraham Solomon, the son of Samuel Solomon, the quack practitioner.

The Wallich family has produced many other notable physicians over the past five centuries. They include the Nobel Prize winner Otto Wallich, as well as Moshe Wallich, founder of the Shaarei Tzedek Hospital in Jerusalem.[6]

However, not all the graduates were bonafide physicians and the successful attempts by various quack doctors in obtaining Aberdeen degrees had important ramifications. They were as aware as genuine practitioners that the degree would enhance their commercial prospects and give their activities an aura of medical legitimacy which sorely tried the universities and medical corporations. Amongst these quacks were two Jewish quack doctors, well known in their day, William Brodum and Samuel Solomon.

William Brodum received his degree on the 15th of January 1791 with affidavits from Dr. Luis Leo, a Jewish practitioner in Houndsditch in London, and a Dr. Saunders who was in the habit of providing recommendations for doctors seeking medical degrees.[7] It was therefore with considerable distress that Marischal College discovered that they had awarded one of their degrees to the 'Empiric Brodum' who was a stall-holder at Covent Garden and was making a fortune from the sales of his Botanical Syrup. Perhaps even more offensive was Brodum's book, *A Guide to Old Age; a Cure for the Indiscretions of Youth*. The introduction was addressed to 'Virgins Uninformed' and contained the necessary, and sexually explicit, information![7]

Marischal College decided to take legal advice and sought the opinion of Mr. Blair, the Solicitor-General for Scotland, on whether it was possible to de-graduate Brodum for 'notorious and impudent quackery....and the immoral tendency of many passages in his various publications.'[8] The Solicitor-General held that it was clear that 'an Incorporation has by law no power to expel its own members.'

Blair considered that, 'The distinction between a Quack, that is to say a person who takes it upon himself to practise physick without having received a proper education and without being graduated Doctor of Medicine, and a regular physician who has been bred to the business and authorised to practise is well known. But amongst those who have received the degree of Doctor of Medicine from a University entitled to grant such degrees (which is the case of Dr. Brodum), I do not know where exactly the line is to be drawn, or what degree of ostentation or ignorance is to fix on a gentleman of this description the imputation of Quackery, so as to afford a legal ground for depriving him of his degree.....The memorialists will consider, therefore, whether under all the circumstances, it may not be most prudent for them to submit in silence as they have hitherto done, to a very unpleasant mortification, and rather if possible to draw good out of evil by making the case of Dr. Brodum a lesson of caution and circumspection to themselves for the future, in bestowing Academical honours.'[8]

As Blair pointed out, the line between quackery and reputable medicine might be difficult to define. After all, Jacob de Castro Sarmento successfully sold his 'Aqua de l'Inglaterra' and his sponsor, and President of the Royal Society, Sir Hans Sloane, was not averse to selling an eye salve. The objection was not the sale of medicine but the pretension of medical expertise inherent in conducting consultations, without a medical training.

The other great Jewish quack of the period was Samuel Solomon, who was born in Cork in 1745, the younger son of Abraham Solomon, who was the shochet, or ritual slaughterer, to the Jewish community there.[9]

There is no doubt that the degrees were of considerable commercial benefit and the two quacks made extensive use of their qualifications. I have been able to identify an advertising campaign by both Solomon and Brodum in the *Glasgow Advertiser*, later known as the *Glasgow Herald*, in 1798.[10] Signifi-

11 Advertisement for the Cordial Balm of Gilead in the *Glasgow Advertiser*, 1798.

cantly, the campaign was aided by John Mennons the founder and first editor of the paper. In the early days the paper was only published twice a week and Mennons looked to avenues outside medicine to augment his income. The various advertisements show that Mennons was not only the printer of works by both Brodum and Solomon but that the medicines could also be obtained from the newspaper offices on appointment. Solomon's *Guide to Health* was as successful a publication as Brodum's *A Guide to Old Age* and ran to many editions.

The advertisements refer to many cures for scurvy, cancer and venereal diseases and authority is lent to their claims of efficacy by their possession of medical qualifications. In one advertisement Solomon styles himself: 'Samuel Solomon M.D. Member of the University and College of Physicians, Aberdeen, &c.&c.'*

It is clear that the medicines of Brodum and Solomon were as successful in Scotland as they were elsewhere.†

Marischal College were undoubtedly mortified by their experience with Brodum and Solomon although it should be noted that they were not the only university to award a degree to the undeserving. The University of Edinburgh had given their M.D. to Sam Leeds, an itinerant brush-maker who had none of the medical pretensions that Brodum and Solomon possessed. Marischal College heeded the advice to be more careful in the future, as the experience of Dr. Hart Wessels shows.

Wessels provided no less than five affidavits for doctors seeking the degree of Doctor of Medicine at Marischal College but after his recommendation of a Dr. Walker, who it transpired was a purveyor of patent medicine, was told that his recommendations would not be accepted in Aberdeen any longer (see Table 3:3—List of Jewish Doctors Providing Attestations for Medical Degrees in Aberdeen).

Wessels wrote back that he had previously given preference to Marischal College but that he would not send them any more applications, and thus the College lost a useful source of revenue which depended on graduation fees from practitioners who had medical sponsors to support them. The Fasti of Marischal College record that Wessels was 'a little doubtful with respect to nostrums but in a great deal of credit as a physician in London.'[11] Marischal College's smooth words were of no avail and Wessels sent them no further applications.

These events illustrate the great desire to have a degree of Doctor of Medicine in the certain expectation that it would improve the status and give the appearance of academic respectability to the commercial aspirations of the quack practitioners. The success of Brodum and Solomon undoubtedly played a part in the greater care that Marischal College took before awarding

---

*Solomon advertised that he left his medicine to the world conscious of having done his 'duty'. 'It may be given ...... with safety and efficacy unknown in the annals of medical discovery'.

†Suppliers were to be found in Glasgow, Edinburgh, Hawick, Stirling and many other parts of Scotland.

Table 3:3 *Jewish Doctors Providing Attestations for Medical Degrees in Aberdeen*

Marischal College		King's College	
Jacob Adolphus	1	Benjamin Lara	1
Philip de la Cour	1	John Meyer	7
Luis Leo	1	Joseph Hart Myers	2
John Meyer	2	Ralph Schomberg	1
Meyer Schomberg	5	Joseph Sequira	1
Hart Wessels	5		

source: Officers and Graduates etc.

their degrees and there is evidence that later applicants were turned down on account of their links with patent medicine. The difficulty in establishing a dividing line between quackery and orthodox practice was confirmed when Brodum successfully sued the Quaker physician John Oakley Lettsom who had hurled a stream of abuse against Brodum in an anti-quack expose.[12]

In the atmosphere of eighteenth century practice, regular practitioners could not yet exert their professional authority. The message was not lost on King's College and the case of Heyman Lion illustrates their desire to award their degree only to reputable physicians irrespective of their medical qualifications.

Lion (c.1760-c.1825) was one of the earliest Jewish residents of Edinburgh, where he was in practice as a dentist and chiropodist. Anxious to improve his status, he enrolled and studied at Edinburgh University between 1790 and 1795, pursuing a regular course of undergraduate studies. He applied for an M.D. in Edinburgh but was turned down by the Senate without any reason being given. He then applied to King's College in Aberdeen where he gave evidence of his undergraduate studies and brought recommendations from Dr. John Barclay, Dr. William Farquharson and Dr. J. Yule. He was again turned down, not because of his qualifications, which were entirely adequate for the degree of M.D., but on account of 'the public line of practice which he has for some time adopted.'[13] In other words, the authorities in neither university were prepared to grant their degree to someone who was engaged in chiropody or dentistry, which was not in keeping with the dignity of Doctor of Medicine. While it might be thought that Lion's European origins told against him, as might his somewhat flamboyant personality, there is not any suggestion that his Jewish background was in itself the cause of his failure to obtain the degree.

Lion returned to his chiropody and was the author of a remarkable 438 page work on the treatment of corns.[14]

While there is little doubt that the awarding of degrees *in absentia* remained a controversial aspect of eighteenth and early nineteenth Scottish medicine, the practice was popular for the mid-career practitioner. Additionally it had the benefit of enabling a number of Jewish doctors to become established as medical graduates. There was a tendency for overseas and provincial Jewish practitioners to receive a recommendation from their local non-Jewish colleagues. For Jewish practitioners in London there was a greater likelihood that affidavits would be received from Jewish colleagues. This suggests that Jewish doctors working abroad or in provincial centres had normal professional contacts with their local non-Jewish medical peers. In London, where there was a larger Jewish medical fraternity, Jewish life could be more cohesive. Similarly, Jewish doctors in London, who were supplying affidavits for Aberdeen diplomas, were more likely to do so for Jewish colleagues while Jewish provinicial doctors had greater professional contacts outwith the community. (Table 3:3)

Graduation *in absentia* could be obtained in St. Andrews as well as in Aberdeen and, as we have seen, the practice continued there longer. However, by the time that Louis Ashenheim graduated in St. Andrews in 1839 it was customary to qualify by examination even though all the medical studies had been conducted elsewhere, often in Edinburgh or London.

Following the graduation of Louis Ashenheim there were four more Jews who graduated there in medicine before 1880. (Table 3:4) The pattern of career choice of these graduates illustrates the problems facing Victorian Jewish doctors. Ashenheim left Scotland, where he had grown up, to settle in Jamaica. Leonard Emanuel, who died at the early age of twenty-nine years, had served in the Indian Army and Simon Belinfante pursued his career in Australia. Alex Zeigler did remain to practise obstetrics in Edinburgh but he, and his son who was an Edinburgh graduate, gradually severed contact with the Jewish community.

Emigration was usually seen as a last resort for Victorian medical men.[15] However, for Jewish practitioners with little chance of patronage in London the more fluid social framework of the colonies, or the possibility of accumulating funds while in the Indian Medical Service, must have seemed a better prospect than joining the ranks of the struggling general practitioners in Britain. Australia was the most popular choice for emigrating doctors from Britain in this period[15] and there were Jews who graduated in Scotland, with Belinfante, Iffla and Louis Ashenheim's brother Charles amongst them.

Among the Jewish medical graduates from St. Andrews it was only Maurice Davis who pursued a career in London. Davis was active within the Jewish community but his medical committee work involved him in the British Medical Association rather than in the more elite medical corporations.

With the increasing reputation of the medical school at Edinburgh University in the last half of the eighteenth century there was attracted to

Table 3:4 Jewish Medical Graduates in St. Andrews Before 1880

1839	Louis Ashenheim
1845	Alexander Zeigler
1852	Maurice Davis
1859	Leonard Emanuel
1862	Simon Belinfante

Edinburgh a large and cosmopolitan student body. One small but significant strand in this student body which came from Britain, Europe, North America and the West Indies, was a number of Jewish students who can be identified from 1767 onwards. (Table 3:5)

The matriculation index at Edinburgh University is comprehensive for the years 1760 to 1860. For the period prior to 1760 it is possible to consult the class lists of William Cullen and Alexander Monro. A detailed index of this nature is not available at the University of Glasgow, where medical students were not required to matriculate before the 1840's. However, study of the material in Glasgow, in the class lists which identify medical students in their various courses between 1800 and 1850, fails to identify positively any Jewish names. When this is compared with the Edinburgh index, in which over twenty Jewish students have been identified, the picture is clear that Edinburgh was the preferred centre of medical studies in this period of almost a hundred years.

Table 3:5 Jewish Medical Students at Edinburgh University Before 1880

		date of studies	qualifications & title of thesis
1.	A.R. Mendes da Costa	1767-8	
2.	Joseph Hart Myers	1775-9	M.D. Edinburgh 'de diabeto'
3.	Levi Myers	1785-8	M.D. Glasgow
4.	Solomon de Leon	1786-8	M.D. Leiden 'de inflammatione'
5.	Moses Nunes Henriques	1789-90	
6.	Joao Pereira de Castro	1790-3	M.D. Edinburgh 'variola'
7.	Heyman Lion	1790-58	
8.	Moses Bravo	1800-1	
9.	Joel Hart	1804-5	LRCS England
10.	Abraham Solomon	1804-10	M.D. Edinburgh 'de cerebri tumoribus'
11.	David Bravo	1808-9	
12.	Miguel Caetano de Castro	1808-11	M.D. Edinburgh 'de aqua frigidae usu'
13.	Alexander Zeigler	1813-16	M.D. St. Andrews
14.	Hananel Mendes da Costa	1815-8	
15.	Hananel de Leon	1816-8	M.D. Edinburgh 'de hydrocephalo'
16.	Joseph Gutteres Henriques	1818-9	
17.	Douglas Cohen	1825-8	M.D. Edinburgh 'de gangrene'
18.	George Charles Wallich	1832-6	M.D. Edinburgh 'on pneumonia'
19.	Aaron Hart David	1834-5	M.D. Edinburgh 'on infanticide'
20.	Louis Ashenheim	1834-7	M.D. St. Andrews
21.	Edwin Adolphus	1834-8	M.D. Edinburgh 'on the pathological characters of urine'
22.	Benjamin Lara	1839-49	
23.	Charles Ashenheim	1843-52	M.D. Edinburgh 'delirium tremens'
24.	Michael Levy	1851-2	
25.	Moritz Stern	1854-9	MRCSE, LRCP London
26.	Henry Fraenkel	1873-8	M.D. Edinburgh
27.	Meyer Bernstein	1874-9	M.D. Edinburgh

source: Matriculation index, Medical Faculty, University of Edinburgh.

That a number of Jewish medical students came to Edinburgh to study in the eighteenth and early nineteenth centuries has never been described before, either in the histories of the Jews in medicine or in Scottish medical histories. This is partly due to the small size of the Jewish community in Scotland in this period, and because the Jewish students were relatively few in number when compared to the very substantial output of the Scottish medical schools.

Precedent had been established in 1739 in Aberdeen when Jacob de Castro Sarmento received the M.D. degree from Marischal College. Precedent was similarly established in Edinburgh in 1767 when the name A.R.M. da Costa (Abraham Raphael Mendes da Costa) appears on the matriculation index for the session 1767-8.

More significant was the graduation, in Edinburgh in 1779, of Joseph Hart Myers (1758-1823), the first Jewish physician to have graduated in Britain after a period of regular undergraduate study.

The minutes of the University for the 15th June, 1779 record a meeting presided over by Professor Black, James Robertson and Dr. Gregory. It was Dr. Gregory who reported from the Faculty of Medicine that a number of students, including Joseph Hart Myers from America, 'had gone through their private briefs with approbation and requested the Senatus Academicus would appoint Wednesday the 24th current for their publick Examination and defending their respective Theses'. The Senatus granted the request and the 24th June was set for the final part of the examination.

At that meeting on June 24th, Principal Robertson was in attendance along with Professor Monro, Professor Black and Professor Hope James Robertson and John Robson were also present and it was recorded that 'the meeting was constituted by prayer by Principal Robertson'. The minutes record that the various candidates 'having gone their several Trials and Examinations and defended their respective Theses' publicly had the degree on M.D. conferred on them. Two other Americans graduated along with Myers and there were five Irish and six English graduates.

Religious tests were not being applied to undergraduates although they had never been formally abolished, and it was thus established that it was possible for Jews in Britain to gain access to a university medical education.

Indeed over the years it is clear that Jews did make use of the spirit of religious and academic freedom available in Scotland. During the early formative years of the Edinburgh Jewish community, between 1775 and 1820, there was hardly a year in which there was not a Jewish medical student enrolled at the University of Edinburgh.

The formation of the Edinburgh Jewish community in 1816 predates that in Glasgow by 7 years. Despite the more rapidly increasing size of the city of Glasgow the two Jewish communities remained quite similar in size over the next forty years, no doubt enhanced by Edinburgh's position on the east coast route for emigration from Europe. Edinburgh also maintained its positive image as virtually the sole centre for Jewish undergraduates in Britain until facilities became available in London with the founding of University College

It has already been noted that it was the 1820's before the Glasgow medical school, with a student population of about 400, began to compete seriously

margin: Degree of MD

and John Robison. The Meeting being constituted by prayer by Principal Robertson, the following gentlemen having gone their several Trials and Examinations and defended their respective Thesis in the publick Hall with the approbation of the Senatus Academicus viz Mr Edward Johnstone from England the subject of whose Thesis is, de Febre puerperale, Mr Arthur Broughton from D° De Vermibus Intestinorum, Mr Gabriel Wynne from D° De Cortice Peruviano usu generis in Morbis febrilibus, Mr Stephen Sellet from D° De Palustrium Locorum insalubritate a Myasmate oriunda, Mr Thomas Waite from D° De Aborta; Mr John Ford from D° De Morbis Contagiosis; Mr William Hamilton from Ireland De Sanguine Humano; Mr Cadwallader Blayney Lee from D° De Rubeola; Mr James Bennett from D° De Hydrope Anasarca; Mr Samuel Hayman from D° De Gastritide; Mr Joseph Hart Myers from America, De Diabete; Mr George Logan from Philadelphia, De Venenis, Mr James Stewart from Maryland De Spasmo had the degree of Doctor of Medicine conferred on them.

Edinr College July 16th 1779.

Present att an University Meeting Principal Robertson, Professor James Robertson, John Robison, Bruce, Dalziel

A Commission from his Majesty was presented to the Principal and Professors by Donald Smith Esqr College Bailie,

margin: Prof. Publick Law

acting by Commission from the Magistrates & Council, to Mr Allan Macconochie Advocate to be Professor of Publick Law and Law of Nature and Nations in this University. The said Commission being presented and read, and found to have passed in due form, they unanimously did admit the said Mr Allan Macconochie to be Professor of Publick Law, and Law of Nature

12   Extract from the Senate Records, University of Edinburgh, 1779, confirming the M.D. degree awarded to Joseph Hart Myers.

DISSERTATIO MEDICA
INAUGURALIS,
DE
DIABETE.
QUAM,
ANNUENTE SUMMO NUMINE,

Ex Auctoritate Reverendi admodum Viri

D. GULIELMI ROBERTSON, S. S. T. P.

ACADEMIÆ EDINBURGENÆ PRÆFECTI;

NEC NON

Ampliſſimi SENATUS ACADEMICI conſenſu,
Et nobiliſſimae FACULTATIS MEDICÆ decreto;

Pro GRADU DOCTORATUS,

SUMMISQUE IN MEDICINA HONORIBUS ET PRIVILEGIIS
RITE ET LEGITIME CONSEQUENDIS;

Eruditorum examini ſubjicit

JOSEPHUS HART MYERS, A. M.

AMERICANUS.

Ad diem 24. Junii, hora locoque ſolitis.

Quo plus ſunt potae, plus ſitiuntur aquae.   OVID.

EDINBURGI:
Apud BALFOUR et SMELLIE,
Academiae Typographos.
M,DCC,LXXIX.

13 Thesis, on diabetes, submitted by Joseph Hart Myers, 1779. Courtesy of Edinburgh University Library.

with Edinburgh. During the eighteenth century the medical school in Glasgow was overshadowed by developments in Edinburgh. At a time when there were regular numbers of Jewish students studying in Edinburgh none can be found in Glasgow until Laurence Joseph commenced his studies there in 1829. While Levi Myers had been the first Jewish graduate at the University of Glasgow, he had not studied there and had taken all his studies in Edinburgh. In fact the first Jewish undergraduate in Glasgow was not a medical student but an American arts student, Marx Cohen (1808-1881).[16] Marx Cohen was the son of Mordecai Cohen, a wealthy English-born southern American with interests in South Carolina and who would have been a contemporary of Levi Myers.

The founding of the Glasgow Hebrew Congregation in 1823 did not prompt the arrival of any further Jewish students in Glasgow. Laurence Alfred Joseph, the first Jewish medical undergraduate in Glasgow, took his M.D. in 1831 after special request, as his regiment, the 4th Dragoon Guards, was due to leave for service in Ireland. Joseph was later known as Dr. Joseph Laurence a name change which he may have employed to try and conceal his Jewish origins.

If a Jew in England wished to graduate in medicine at university in the eighteenth or early nineteenth century the options were strictly limited. Such qualifications could only be obtained in Scotland or at one of the continental universities, usually in Holland or Germany. In 1840 the famous Jewish pharmacologist Jonathan Pereira decided to leave his post, as Professor of Materia Medica at the Aldersgate Medical School to become a candidate for the post of assistant physician at the London Hospital.[17] At first, he planned to leave London for a couple of years to come to Scotland, presumably to study in Edinburgh. However, he changed his plans and took the qualifications of the licentiate of the Royal College of Physicians of London. He then obtained the degree of M.D. from Erlangen in Bavaria and was elected to the post he sought. He had reached the position of Professor of Materia Medica with the license of the Society of Apothecaries but he could not, as a Jew, graduate at a university in England.

However, given the small size of Anglo-Jewry in the eighteenth century recruitment of Jewish students to the Scottish universities was from a wide geographical area. In fact, for much of the period overseas students predominated, with the number of British Jews only beginning to increase as the Jewish population of Britain expanded during the nineteenth century.

Many of the first Jewish graduates hailed from America. They included Joseph Hart Myers as well as Levi Myers and Joel Hart. Levi Myers, who was not related to Joseph Hart Myers, graduated in Glasgow at the end of his second year of studies in Edinburgh after giving evidence of his undergraduate work. He returned to Edinburgh for a third year of studies and matriculated as Dr. Levi Myers M.D. (Glas.).

Joel Hart was born in Philadelphia in 1784 and studied medicine in both London and Edinburgh being a matriculated student at the University of Edinburgh for the 1804-5 session.[18] He returned to the United States after becoming a licentiate of the Royal College of Surgeons of England and was one of the charter members of the Medical Society of the County of New York.

A high proportion of the Jewish students who came to study in Edinburgh hailed from the West Indies. Indeed, with the exception of Solomon de Leon who came from the island of St. Kitts, all the Jewish West Indians hailed from Jamaica. Jews settled on Jamaica early in colonial times with groups of Jews from England and South America reaching the island from the 1660's. While the full franchise was not granted until 1831 the Jews achieved a high measure of emancipation in the eighteenth century and this, allied to a high level of material prosperity, created the right conditions to attract members of the community into the professions. Scotland was the principal source for foreign medical students from the West Indies from the late eighteenth century and a number of Jews can be identified amongst the West Indian medical students in Scotland.

The Jewish community on Jamaica has never been very large, peaking at about 2,500 souls in the 1880's when with declining prosperity many Jews left the island to settle in United States and Britain.

The first Jew to come from Jamaica to study in Scotland was Moses Nunes Henriques who matriculated for one session at Edinburgh University in 1789-1790. There were a number of Jamaican Jewish families with the surname Henriques and there is a particularly close link between the Henriques and the Scottish medical schools which has continued into modern times. Ernest, the son of Nathaniel Henriques, of Kingston, Jamaica came to Aberdeen to study, graduating M.D. there in 1898 and settling to practise in Lancashire. His daughter Stella also studied in Aberdeen, graduating M.B. Ch.B. there in 1923, although by this time that branch of the family had severed all connection with Jewish life. In 1933 Horace Leslie Cohen Henriques graduated M.B. Ch.B. in Glasgow and in 1960 the first Jewish woman from Jamaica to graduate in medicine, Marilyn Alberga, whose mother was a Henriques, did so at the University of Glasgow. This custom of successive generations finding their way back to the medical schools frequented by parents and teachers is a recurring one in medical history and the story of Jamaican Jews studying medicine in Scotland is therefore almost two hundred years long.

Most of the Jamaican Jews studied only briefly in Edinburgh, usually only for one academic year, although Hananel de Leon studied for two years in Edinburgh graduating there in 1818 and Moritz Stern spent five years in Edinburgh from 1854. The Edinburgh experience was therefore part of a general medical education which could be selected by the student and which would equip the aspiring practitioner for his future career. This is well illustrated by the medical career of Joseph Gutteres Henriques. He was born in Jamaica in 1796 and came to Britain to study medicine, at first entering St. Thomas's Hospital in London.[19] There he won a considerable number of prizes and he is said to have been a favourite pupil of Sir Astley Cooper and Sir William Lawrence. After two years in London, Henriques came to Edinburgh and enrolled at Edinburgh University for the 1818-1819 session. Henriques never managed to become Consultant Physician at the Finsbury Hospital due, he thought, to anti-Jewish prejudice, and he subsequently retired from medical practice to concentrate on Jewish communal work. Other Jamaican Jews studying medicine in Edinburgh included David and Moses Bravo, who practised in Jamaica.

The Jamaican link was not solely confined to Jamaican natives coming to Scotland to study, for there was an emigration of Jewish doctors to Jamaica. As we have seen, Judah Israel Montefiore, who graduated at King's College, Aberdeen, settled in Jamaica as did, for a while, Solomon Iffla, the first Jewish licentiate at the Faculty of Physicians and Surgeons in Glasgow. Jews were thus being attracted to Scotland, to study medicine, from England, North America and the West Indies. From about 1840 there came an increasing number of South Africans. During colonial times Edinburgh was the most popular choice for all South Africans studying medicine, even among those of Dutch descent. Jewish South Africans followed this trend with the first South African of Jewish origin to qualify in medicine in Scotland, Henry Fraenkel, who qualified at Edinburgh University in 1878. The Fraenkel family had a long history of medical practice in South Africa. The founder was a German Jew, Seigried Fraenkel, who settled at the Cape in 1808 and was one of the earliest Jewish residents there,[20] and his son carried on the tradition.

There was an early tradition of Jews in medicine in South Africa fostered by a group of German Jewish doctors from Hesse-Cassel who settled around Graaff-Reinet after 1840.[21] These Jewish doctors brought culture and stability to this area of Cape Colony and constituted the advance guard of Jewish practitioners in South Africa. They integrated well with the local communities and enhanced the status of Jewish doctors among the local Afrikaaners. Among their descendents were medical students who came to Scotland to study.

South Africans continued to come to Scotland in significant numbers until well into the twentieth century as the first medical schools did not develop there until 1912. Edinburgh continued to attract more South Africans than the other Scottish medical schools and there was a South African Students' Union there until 1936.

Jewish students were well represented among the South Africans studying in Scotland, with their proportion reaching almost one third between the World Wars, although South African Jewry never exceeded 5% of the white population. By 1927 there were 392 Jewish doctors in South Africa who formed over 19% of the local medical profession.[22] South African Jewry shared the same geographical roots as Scottish Jewry and were overwhelmingly of Lithuanian origin. However, the Jews in South Africa managed to enter medicine in large numbers from the turn of the century while Scottish Jews did not achieve this until after the First World War.

The Jewish South Africans identified strongly with Jewish life while studying in Scotland and made an important contribution to Jewish life on the campuses, especially in Edinburgh where they dominated Jewish student activities until the 1930's.[23] A majority of the South Africans who qualified in Scotland returned home to practise but a number stayed on in Britain. In time they were joined by Jewish doctors who had qualified in South Africa and came to Britain to find work. Studying in Edinburgh proved to be a valuable help in the conduct of a medical career even if it was not always accompanied by obtaining the Edinburgh M.D. While it might be more difficult for Jewish practitioners to become established in the more competitive areas of medical practice, particularly where the jurisdiction of the Royal College ran, for overseas Jewish practitioners returning home the advantages were clear. Moritz Stern, who studied in Edinburgh in the 1850's, returned to Jamaica where he became surgeon to the Militia and President of the Jamaican branch of the British Medical Society.[24]

Prominent amongst overseas physicians who studied and graduated in Edinburgh was Aaron Hart David (1812-1882) who was born in Montreal.[25,26] David was proud of his connections with Scotland and was able to carry the Edinburgh tradition to Montreal, a city where standards from the inception of medical education were based on those achieved in Edinburgh. Scots born Jews began to study at university and to graduate with Louis Ashenheim who had been born in Edinburgh in 1816 the son of Jacob Ashenheim, a jeweller who had emigrated from Holland to Scotland. Jacob Ashenheim had prospered in Edinburgh and was able to provide his children with a university education. Louis Ashenheim entered Edinburgh University in 1834 and studied there for three years, although he graduated in St. Andrews. Ashenheim was a noted writer as well as a physician and he spent some time in London before leaving for Jamaica in 1843.[27]

Louis Ashenheim's younger brother Charles (1828-1866) was also a medical student at Edinburgh University with a long undergraduate career between 1843 and 1852, although with a couple of interruptions. He obtained the license of the Royal College of Surgeons of Edinburgh before finally returning to Edinburgh University in 1851 and he was awarded his M.D. degree in 1852 with a thesis on 'delirium tremens'. Charles Ashenheim was obviously a less assiduous student than his older brother and it is interesting to note that Michael Levy was a matriculated student at Edinburgh University in 1851-2. Levy was Ashenheim's brother-in-law and one wonders whether he had enrolled at university to keep a close eye on the wayward student who was taking so long to obtain his qualifications!

Virtually all of the Jewish students, identified as studying in Edinburgh, did so at the University. At the beginning of the nineteenth century it was still quite common to obtain a medical education by apprenticeship to an established physician and although the practice was much less common during the 1830's it did not become obsolete until about 1850. It is likely that the Manchester Jewish physician Isaac Abraham Franklin undertook a medical apprenticeship in Edinburgh as his name does not appear on the matriculation roll at Edinburgh University. The records of the Royal College of Surgeons of England show that Franklin became a Licentiate of the Society of Apothecaries of London in 1834 and a Member of the Royal College of Surgeons in 1835. It is noted there that he had studied in Manchester and in Edinburgh. Franklin became one of the leading medical men in Manchester and remained an active and devout member of the Manchester Jewish community and was typical of the new Anglo-Jewish bourgeoisie which sought adaptation to British society allied to uncompromising loyalty to traditional Jewish practices. Thus, the history of Jews in medicine in Britain from earliest times illustrates the effects of academic emancipation. For some, like Franklin, Myers, Davis and Joseph Hart, medical education enabled them to take their place both in Jewish and the wider society while for the Zeiglers and Charles Ashenheim the way led directly out of the Jewish community.[28]

Thus there were many options available for the Jewish doctor in terms of their role within the Jewish community, but the choices were more restricted in the pursuit of their professional goals. The Jewish medical students in Edinburgh were not the leading members of the British medical profession. Within a society that was largely Anglican and Anglo-Saxon, Jewish practitioners might have expected to have some initial difficulties in reaching the heights of the medical profession. The ties of ethnic and religious affiliation could also work to the advantage of Jewish practitioners as Meyer Schomberg discovered at an early stage.[29] Schomberg cultivated the Jews of the Ashkenazi Dukes Place Synagogue thereby building up a prosperous clientele which enabled him to become one of the best paid physicians of his day. A few Jewish doctors were able to base their clientele almost entirely within the confines of the Jewish community and this occurred also with other minority groups such as the Catholics.[30]

There were many problems involved in setting up in practice. Money was needed to establish the practitioner and patronage was essential to enter the hospital service and to attempt to enter the ranks of the professional elites. The Jewish practitioners therefore turned their attentions in other directions. They achieved distinction overseas, especially in the West Indies and in Australia, and were well regarded in medicine in the provinces. Franklin practised in Manchester, Douglas Cohen in Liverpool and Benjamin Lara continued the medical traditions of his family in Portsmouth. Joseph Hart Myers, Solomon de Leon and Hananel de Leon settled in London, but with much of their practice as physicians to the Hebra, and thus within the Jewish community.

Despite this, Edinburgh University performed a vital role for Jewish students. For almost a hundred years it was the only British university which admitted Jewish students and it had done so long before the final drama of the Jewish emancipation movement. Jews were keen to enter medicine and Edinburgh offered the path into the profession. While other doors were barred, enough Jewish medical students came to Edinburgh to disprove suggestions that Jews were not well represented in medicine in Britain in the eighteenth and early nineteenth centuries or that Jews had not taken advantage of the attractions and freedoms of Scottish medicine.

Within Scotland the first Jewish students had mixed fortunes, Heyman Lion ended his student days no doubt bitterly frustrated by the experience. Both Louis and Charles Ashenheim emigrated and the Zeiglers advanced within Edinburgh, both medically and socially, at the expense of their Jewish origins.

We turn now to consider Scottish Jews in medicine amongst whom the best known was Asher Asher (1837-1889).[31,32] He was born in Glasgow, the son of immigrants from the Polish city of Lublin, and was a pupil at the High School of Glasgow. From his earliest days he proved to be an assiduous scholar of Hebrew and the Bible and he was a skilled linguist. His father never

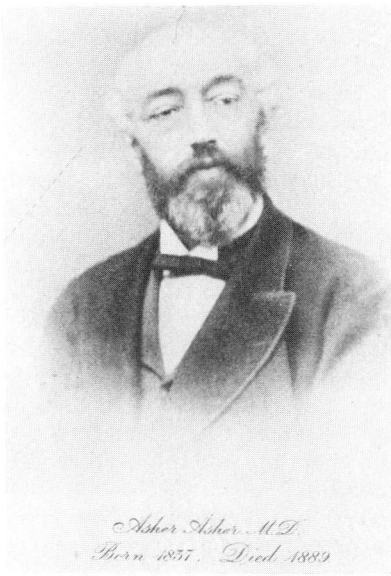

14 Asher Asher, physician in Glasgow and London.

advanced far materially but was a Hebrew scholar in his own right and gave his son a good grounding in these subjects.[33] He supported himself as an undergraduate by working as a bookkeeper in a local Jewish firm and proved to be a good student, winning a class prize in materia medica and taking first place in the class of forensic medicine. He graduated from Glasgow University in 1855 and in the following year became a licentiate of the Royal College of Surgeons of Edinburgh. (Tables 3:6 and 3:7)

Dr. Asher began to practise in Bishopbriggs, then a colliery town near Glasgow. Despite the poor income offered by the Parochial Boards the majority of those employed as Medical Officers were, like Asher Asher, university graduates who would have looked on their work as the first rung in their

Table 3:6 *Jewish Medical Graduates at the University of Glasgow Before 1880*

Levi Myers	1787
Laurence Alfred Joseph	1831
Joseph Marcus Joseph	1852 (Ll.D. 1866)
Asher Asher	1855
Samuel Levenston	1859
Reuben Gross	1862

source: Graduation Album of the University of Glasgow, 1727-1897 (Glasgow, 1897).

Table 3:7   Jewish Licentiates of the Royal College of Surgeons of Edinburgh

1.	Aaron Hart David, M.D. Edin.	1834
2.	George Charles Wallich, M.D. Edin.	1837
3.	Louis Ashenheim, M.D. St. A.	1840
4.	Charles Ashenheim, M.D. Edin.	1848
5.	Asher Asher, M.D. Glas.	1856
6.	Reuben Gross, M.D. Glas.	1862

source: List of licentiates of the Royal College of Surgeons of Edinburgh.

medical career. The position of Medical Officer gave the doctor access to the committee of management and gave him much necessary experience in his initial medical career.

When Asher settled in London he worked initially with Dr. Jacob Canstatt who was a general practitioner in the East End of London and who had in 1859 taken over the responsibility of the medical care of the Jewish poor in London. This care had previously been undertaken by the major London synagogues and was now the responsibility of the London Jewish Board of Guardians. Asher's previous experience in Cadder, along with his fluency in English, Hebrew and Yiddish, would have been considerable assets in his new work.

Asher was greatly missed in Glasgow. He had served as Honorary Secretary of the Glasgow Hebrew Congregation from 1860 to 1862 and he continued to pursue his studies in Hebrew language and Jewish religious lore, a field in which he exhibited deep erudition and in which he had been almost entirely self-taught.

The annual reports of the Jewish Board of Guardians, now known as the Jewish Welfare Board, for the period 1862 to 1866 were written by Asher Asher and they clearly illustrate the efficient manner in which his new duties were conducted. Careful guidelines were set down for the work and ample statistics were printed permitting audit of the activities undertaken. The functioning of the new medical service was monitored monthly and the reports served to furnish a guide to the miserable living conditions of the time. Malnutrition, poor housing and a lack of sanitation characterised the way of life of London's Jewish, and non-Jewish poor.

In his first report, Dr. Asher pointed out the factors which operated to the detriment of health and caused the destruction of the lives of members of the Jewish community, these being lack of food and clothing, lack of facilities for cleaning, poor ventilation, overcrowding and deficient light. Asher made strenuous efforts to combat these problems, playing a small part in trying to reverse the ravages of chronic poverty. Convalescent care was organised, coal and blankets were provided and with cleaning facilities provided, a pride in hygiene was manifested. In his second report he was pleased to note that the number of fevers (typhus and others) had dropped from 383 to 206 with the number of deaths reduced from 10 to 5.

Table 4:1   Growth of Scottish Jewry

Year	Glasgow	Edinburgh	Aberdeen	Dundee
1831	47	50	—	—
1850	150	150	—	—
1880	1,500	500	—	50
1897	4,000	1,000	50	150
1905	6,500	1,200	70	150
1921	13,000	1,800	100	150
1935	15,000	2,000	100	150

source: prior to 1880 from Cecil Roth, *Rise of Provincial Jewry* (1951) after 1880 from *Jewish Year Books*

Scotland by the growth of the cotton industry and the need to escape from poverty and famine.[3] During the same period there were many Highlanders arriving in Glasgow following their displacement from the land during the Highland Clearances. The Gaels formed their own sub-group in urban Scotland, based on language and religion, which encouraged their cohesion as a minority group in the English speaking areas of Scotland.[4] Like these other minority groups the Jews hoped to preserve their distinctive way of life while participating to the full in the commercial, professional and cultural life of their new country.

The growth of the Jewish community was slow during the first decades after the establishment of the Jewish communities in Edinburgh and Glasgow. At first there were more Jewish immigrants from Germany and Holland but very soon the Eastern European element predominated and by 1881, when the major exodus from Eastern Europe was only just getting under way, a census in the Glasgow Jewish community showed that three quarters of the community, then numbering less than 2,000 souls, were of Polish origins.[5] This confirms the findings in Manchester that the ethnic composition of the Jewish community after 1880 did not differ so much from the pre-1880 element as is often believed.[6]

The large majority of the new Jewish immigrants came from historical Lithuania which included large parts of Russia, Latvia and Poland. The proximity of these Jewish communities to the Baltic ports made emigration easier during time of stress. The Jewish Lithuanian, or Litvak, was looked on, and certainly regarded himself, as more enlightened and progressive than his Eastern European brethren and the possessor of a sharper mind.[7] He was more worldly and less influenced by the pietistic Chassidic movement.

In the early and middle nineteenth century the predominant Jewish commercial interest in Scotland was centred in Dundee. From about 1840 Jewish agents from Hamburg, and other parts of Germany, moved into Dundee for the purchase of cheap linens and packing cloths.[8] By the 1850's Jewish firms in Hamburg were sending representatives to Dundee and within a generation they were making their mark on the social and commerical life of the city.

The newcomers from Germany quickly assimilated, a number actually converted to Christianity and no Jewish community was formed in Dundee until 1874.[9]

The small number of Jews already settled in Scotland was completely overwhelmed by the flood of Jewish emigrants from Eastern Europe after 1880. Millions of Jews were on the move westwards following the passage of the restrictive May Laws in 1882 and the regular occurrences of brutal pogroms. The flood, which was mainly directed towards America, could not be contained. The small acculturated groups of Scottish Jews which had grown slowly during the century were quickly outnumbered by a large influx of Yiddish speaking newcomers. This influx changed the nature of Jewish life in Scotland profoundly.

There were many responses to the flood of destitute Jews arriving in Britain after 1880. Many wished to travel onwards to the United States and they were given assistance to do so. Others managed to settle in Britain but attempts were also made within the Jewish community to stem the flow of arrivals. Appeals were made to Jewish leaders in Russia to encourage their communities to stay where they were and not to swell the ranks of impoverished Jews in Britain.[10]* Repatriation was organised by the Glasgow Jewish Board of Guardians but the numbers were very small and it was emphasised that this was only done as a last resort and with the full consent of those concerned.[11] In addition help was given to enable Jewish travellers to re-unite with their families in America. A fund was set up in Glasgow during the First World War to enable consumptives to settle in warmer climates and assistance was given after the War to stateless Jews resident in Glasgow who wished to travel on to the United States.

The influx of immigrants slowed considerably after the passage of the Aliens Act in 1905, a measure which did not find much favour in the Glasgow Jewish community.[12] Apart from a small group of immigrants after the First World War further numerical growth, until the 1930's, came about by natural increase. From 1933 over one thousand central European refugees settled in Scotland. Glasgow Jewry was quick to raise funds for refugee relief: they organised foster homes for displaced children, a hostel for temporary accommodation and attempted to find work to integrate the newcomers. Most of the refugees who came to Scotland settled in Glasgow and in Edinburgh, with only a few outside the two main cities. The new refugees had much to contribute to the Jewish community and to Scotland as a whole. Initially there was a warm welcome but with the approach of war all foreigners were treated with a degree of suspicion and some were actually interned at the outset of war.

Within Glasgow Jewry there was some acrimony over the handling of refugee funds and there was a general feeling that the refugees were not attending synagogue and that the most successful ones were not giving

---

*The London Jewish Board of Guardians organised the return of some 50,000 Jewish men, women and children to Eastern Europe between 1880 and 1914.

sufficient support to communal charities.[13]. However, as the war progressed the two groups came together especially as the newcomers became more proficient in English and more familiar with community norms. Thus, by the end of the war the refugees were, on the whole, well integrated.

That the large majority of Jews settling in Scotland after 1880 chose Glasgow as their destination confirms Glasgow's position at the time as the leading centre in Scotland for commerce and industry. Glasgow provided opportunities in the clothing, furniture and tobacco industries and there was the chance of economic and social advance. The newcomers benefitted from the experience of the Jews who were already settled into the life of the city. Glasgow Jewry had become well respected thanks to the efforts of those like Michael Simons, a Glasgow baillie who was a successful fruit broker and played a prominent part in Jewish life, and the Davis family, present in the city from the founding of the community in 1823 and well known for their generous donations to city hospitals.[14] Close links between Jew and Gentile extended into social contacts and it was reported positively that the majority of the guests at the Glasgow Hebrew Philanthropic Society Ball in 1878 were non-Jews.[15]

The Glasgow Jewish community began to grow after 1870 when there were still only about 40 Jewish families in the city. By 1875 it was accepted that there was a need for a new synagogue and in 1879 the Glasgow Hebrew Congregation moved from George Street to the large and handsome building in Garnethill which cost the substantial sum of £14,000 to build. The style and scale of the building suggests a stable and prosperous community.

The Jewish community in Edinburgh was also considerably augmented by the Eastern European immigration. Most of the Edinburgh community arrived through the port of Leith, some having first docked at Hull or Dundee, but others came as groups to work in various factories. One group from Manchester transferred their activities in the developing waterproofing industry to Edinburgh working for the Caledonian Rubber Company, and establishing a synagogue in Caledonia Crescent in the Dalry district of the city.[16] Other groups of Jews came from Leeds to work in the slipper factory in Guthrie Street, where one of the rooms was fitted out as a synagogue, and from London in 1902 attracted north by the opportunities for work during a strike of Edinburgh tailors.[17]

Over one and a half million Jews travelled across Britain in one of the various trans-shipment routes. They usually preferred, for financial reasons, to cross the North Sea to Hull and then cross England to sail to America from Liverpool, rather than make the Atlantic crossing directly from Hamburg. Not all the travellers reached America and some dropped out at the various Jewish communities which grew up in the towns along the Hull-Liverpool railway line. A smaller number of passengers reached Scotland in this way arriving in Leith or Dundee. In July 1891 a group of transmigrants arriving in Leith were in a 'wretched state' and were supplied with food before they travelled to Glasgow. A further group in October of that year were barely able to fast on Yom Kippur. Scottish Jewry was considerably invigorated by the arrival of those who felt that they had travelled far enough or who believed, or were tricked into believing, that they had already reached America![18] In addition to the Jews in transit Scottish Jewry benefitted from the arrival of Jews from England in search of employment. There were such groups coming to Glasgow in addition to those, as we have seen, which settled in Edinburgh. Jacob Kramrisch brought 300 workers, most of whom were Jewish, to Glasgow in 1888 to manufacture cigarettes for the Imperial Tobacco Company[19] and there were also other smaller groups.

Glasgow Jewry numbered 4,000 by 1897 and almost doubled again in the next five years.[20,21] Almost as soon as the new groups of immigrants arrived a series of mutual aid societies and welfare systems were organised to cater for the needs of the time. These societies showed the ability of Scottish Jewry to establish organisations capable of dealing with the needs of its weaker members. They underlined the determination of the Jews to defend their community and improve its status. In addition to the purely welfare considerations this aided the cohesion of the community and promoted the idea in the wider community that the Jews looked after the needs of their own needy co-religionists. There were Jewish aid societies to support the destitute newcomers though facilities, such as those provided by the Board of Guardians,* were being overwhelmed after 1886.[22] Between 1891 and 1892 the Board of Guardians case-load increased by one-third and they had to seek aid from the Russian Jewish Relief Fund in London. In May 1897 a Jewish Strangers' Aid Society was founded in Glasgow which provided hospitality and welcoming support from its centre in the Gorbals where the new Jewish immigrants were settling. As many as 685 refugees were sheltered in 1905 for an average stay of 7 days and a similar institution in Edinburgh, the Jewish House of Refuge, sheltered 124 people in 1910.[23,24]

The rapid growth of Scottish Jewry matched the increase in the Anglo-Jewish community as a whole. The main aim of the Jews leaving Eastern Europe was to reach the United States of America, popularly referred to in Yiddish as 'di goldeneh medina', (the golden land).

The Glasgow Hebrew Boot and Clothing Guild was formed in 1905 to supply footwear and clothing to the needy and it also co-operated with the Glasgow Corporation Education Department in providing annual holidays for 'necessitous children'. In the 1890's the Philanthropic Society became known as the Jewish Board of Guardians and in 1925 its headquarters moved to 52 Thistle Street in the Gorbals. The work from this centre was continuous. In 1918 they distributed 2 tons of matzot and 1 ton of potatoes for Passover and in the light of social conditions during the 1930's an unemployment bureau was set up.[25] The Glasgow Hebrew Benevolent Loan Society was founded in 1888 to provide interest free loans to members of the community who required temporary financial assistance or who were looking for aid in becoming financially independent.[26] Similar enterprises were formed in Edinburgh and Dundee. The Glasgow society began as the 'penny society' as subscribers paid 1d weekly and in 1899 £57 out of the total income of £92 was subscribed

---

*Originally founded as the Glasgow Hebrew Philanthropic Society in 1858.

in penny shares.[27] The scale of the operation subsequently increased and it was estimated by 1937 that upwards of £80,000 had been granted in loans since 1888.

A Welfare Clinic and Dispensary was founded in 1911 at 11 Apsley Place with Dr. Saul Harris as its medical officer.[28] This clinic was run under the auspices of the Jewish Board of Guardians who aimed to combat the problem of poor Jews being enticed into the well-equipped dispensaries of the Christian missionaries who used welfare facilities as a cover for conversionist activities.[28] The Clinic and Dispensary were subsequently moved to larger premises in Abbotsford Place where preventive medical care and child and maternal health provision was on hand. Poor hospitalised immigrants were also the target for the missionaries and a Jewish Sick Visiting Association was founded in 1899 to visit Jewish patients and a kosher kitchen was provided at the Southern General Hospital in Glasgow.[29]

The various missionary groups saw the presence of large Jewish groups in Glasgow and Edinburgh as a considerable challenge. There had been missionary activity in Glasgow from 1884 and a Missionary Vigilance Society was set up in 1894. The provision of facilities by Christian missionaries for the Jewish community undoubtedly stimulated improvements in Jewish welfare services. The missionary societies were unable to claim many converts, however, and in 1906 the Glasgow Jewish Evangelical Mission reported that they had spent £181 in relief to the Jews but that the results of the Mission should not be judged by the paucity of converts.[30] Leon Levison ran the Edinburgh Medical Mission to the Jews which supplied medical aid and evangelical teaching. Levison's attempts to pose as the benefactor of the Jews caused considerable resentment and his receipt of a knighthood for services to the Russian Jewish Relief Fund was condemned within the Jewish community as the 'prostitution of honours'.[31]

The social cohesion of the community was aided by the formation of a network of friendly societies both in Edinburgh and in Glasgow. With their colourful rituals and uniforms they helped to bring some cheer into many otherwise drab lives. These societies had their own sick visitors, loan and welfare activities. Membership of these societies often reflected the *landsmanschaft* links fostered by immigrant groups from the same small East European towns, or shtetls. In 1922 the Jewish friendly societies in Glasgow and Edinburgh sponsored a convalescent house at Slamannan, near Falkirk, but its closure only three years later was partially blamed on the underfunding of the societies whose total income in 1925 was only £80.[32,33] There was also the Unity Lodge which operated out of 150 Gorbals Street where the Workers' Circle was based. The Workers' Circle had both trade union and friendly society elements and a branch of the United Garment Workers Union was run from its premises. It gave support to left-wing groups and in the 1930's supported the socialists in Spain and Germany.

Union activities were hard to organise given the small size of the sweated workshops and the desperate need for work. This led to undoubted exploitation in the proliferating small workrooms in the Gorbals. However, there were none of the complaints about Jewish landlordism which plagued the

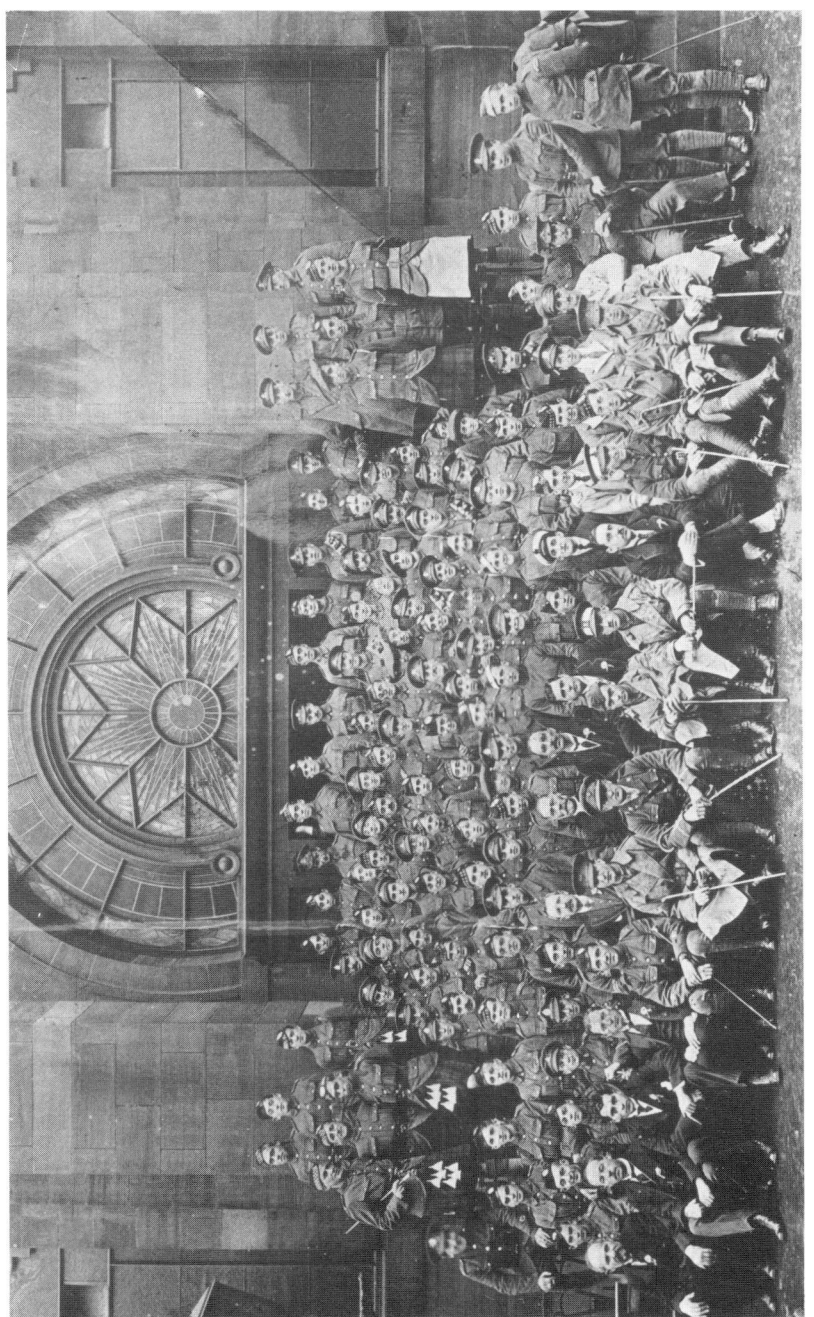

15 Scots like any other! Jewish servicemen gather outside the synagogue, South Portland Street, Glasgow in 1917.

immigrant areas of Leeds. A Glasgow Jewish Socialist League was formed in 1934 to promote Jewish and socialist aims in the general and Jewish communities.[34]

Institutional care in the pre-1939 period consisted mainly of the Gertrude Jacobson Orphanage which was established in 1913 and moved to larger premises in Sinclair Drive in 1919. Some refugee children were also accommodated in addition to orphaned Jewish children from the various communities in Scotland. Besides the shortlived Slamannan convalescent home there were two unsuccessful attempts to set up an old age home, firstly in a tenement flat in Nicolson Street in the Gorbals in 1913 and again in 1929 when a house was purchased in Dixon Avenue.[35]

Societies were also formed to assist the newcomers in becoming British subjects which would reduce the alien character of the community. Jewish Naturalisation Societies were formed in Glasgow and Edinburgh in 1897 and gave advice in Yiddish and enabling the reduced legal fees to be paid for at the rate of one shilling weekly.[36,37] An advertisement in the Glasgow Yiddish Evening Times of 1914 shows the Glasgow Jewish Naturalisation Society, under the aegis of one of the Jewish Friendly Societies, appealing to the public to become naturalised. It emphasised that it was important to cease being strangers and to become English subjects. The concept of being Scottish did not develop until a later date[38] and the Garnethill and Graham Street Synagogues, where the more assimilated Jews gathered were known as the 'English shuls'.

There was also a network of social groupings which aided the cohesion of the growing Glasgow community by providing a framework for activities which was not purely religious. These were usually established first north of the river where the more acculturated Jews, who were often members of the Garnethill Synagogue, were to be found. This suggests that these groups were intended to show that the integration of Jews into Scottish life did not mean the abandonment of Jewish culture but that these ideals could be preserved in a Jewish setting. In an environment where religious traditionalism was on the decline, Scottish Jewry found ways of expressing their social cohesion amid growing acculturation by the forming of organisations in which these aims would be enhanced.

Glasgow had Jewish Workingmen's Clubs on both sides of the river in the 1880's and further groups developed over the years. The Jewish Literary Society was founded in 1893 and promoted Jewish culture in an English format. One of the most successful societies was the Glasgow Jewish Institute whose origins can be traced back to 1900. It achieved its greatest success when it moved to specially adapted premises adjacent to the South Portland Street Synagogue in 1935 where it formed one of the community pivots. Its members excelled in bridge, chess and the dramatic arts and by 1937 its membership was close to 2,300.[39] The Jewish Institute Players, whose origins go back to the founding of the Jewish Dramatic Society in 1905, flourished under the direction of their gifted founder Avrom Greenbaum, after whom the company is now named. Greenbaum was pre-occupied with man's fight for freedom and the Players' repertoire reflected this. The Players had a link with the Unity Theatre, the great people's theatre of the period. The community also maintained choirs and supported the visit of travelling Yiddish plays and artists. In the visual arts the talents of Benno Schotz were recognised as early as 1921 when Schotz exhibited his bust of Theodor Herzl.[40]

In Edinburgh, too, a considerable number of social groups were formed. In the early years of the twentieth century there was a Jewish Amateur Orchestral Society. The Edinburgh Jewish Amateur Dramatic Society was already in existance in 1909 when they performed a Yiddish play and they continued to stage performances through the 1930's. The community also had a Jewish Institute and one of the most enduring of the Edinburgh societies has been the Jewish Literary Society which was formed in 1888. It consistently provided a platform for Jewish subjects within the community and was able to attract some who were not affiliated to the synagogue. It was carefully nurtured by Rabbi Daiches and it is now the oldest society of its kind in Britain.

The Glasgow Jewish Representative Council was formed early in 1914 eight years after the break up of the United Synagogue which had linked Garnethill and some of the Gorbals community. Gorbals Jewry had formed the Jewish Communal Council in 1907 to look after religious matters and to appoint a Rabbi for the Gorbals community. The catalyst to the founding of the Representative Council was the need to protest about the 'blood libel' trial of Mendel Beilis in Kiev[41] but other problems quickly followed. The immediate concerns of the Glasgow Jewish Representative Council were to bring about order in the provision of Kosher meat and to improve Jewish education by establishing a Jewish day school. During the War the Council provided registration for Jews who did not hold British citizenship and obtained the release of 25 interned Jews. The formation of the Council marked the realisation that Jewish rights were more than the provision of welfare, educational and religious services and gave the Jewish community a voice on matters of national and international importance. A Jewish Representative Council was formed in Edinburgh in 1916 but with the formation of the Edinburgh Hebrew Congregation in 1920 this body assumed the function of representing the community to the outside world.

As the Jewish community in Glasgow continued to grow south of the river Clyde it was felt that the Garnethill Synagogue was rather inaccessible to the newcomers and new synagogues were established in the Gorbals. The first Gorbals congregation in Main Street came under the jurisdiction of Garnethill in 1884 but other groups also developed. The Chevra Kadisha Congregation was founded in 1889 and the Great Synagogue in South Portland Street was opened in 1901. Traditional religious practice in Glasgow was centred there under the leadership of Benjamin Atlas who was Rabbi for over thirty years from the end of the First World War. During this period the synagogue was visited regularly by religious luminaries from Eastern Europe who came to pray, lecture, exhort and raise funds for institutions back home. It housed the Glasgow Yeshiva and Mikva and was a place of constant learning and prayer. In 1901 also the Beth Medrash Hagodol was founded in Oxford Street and later, as the New Central Synagogue, moved to Hospital Street in 1925.

Many of the new Gorbals prayer-houses had the small, homely atmosphere typical of the Orthodoxy of Eastern Europe which preferred the small conventicle, or shteible, to the larger and more formal houses of worship. Groups of worshippers from places like Odessa and Minsk founded their own minyanim, or prayer groups, and there was also a small Chassidic group, the Nusach Ari, which existed until about 1930.

In Edinburgh, the old synagogue in Park Place, which had been in use since 1868, had gradually decayed and was surrounded by university buildings. A new building, an old chapel, in Graham Street was acquired in 1896 and opened for Jewish worship two years later. The Graham Street Synagogue was enlarged in 1913 and served as the main Edinburgh synagogue until the present building in Salisbury Road was opened in 1932.

The Rev. Jacob Furst served as minister in Graham Street from 1879 till shortly before his death in 1918. At first he must have preached in Yiddish as a suggestion was made in 1901 that he be allowed to deliver a lecture in English on special occasions.[42]

In the early years of the twentieth century a Jewish prayer house was formed in the Glasgow southern districts of Govanhill (1901). Synagogues were established in Queens Park (1906) and Langside (1916) and these congregations erected larger buildings later. Communities were established in Pollokshields in 1929 and in Giffnock and Newlands in 1938. A synagogue was founded in Crosshill in 1932 which was known as the 'cut-price shul' as subscriptions did not exceed one shilling per week. A community was established also in South West Glasgow based in Hillington, Mosspark and Cardonald, but it never achieved the size to build a synagogue and it gradually dissolved during the 1950's. The amount of new synagogue building between the wars caused some anxiety as Glasgow's synagogues were not all filled on a Saturday morning and some of the older synagogues, especially the Great Synagogue in South Portland Street, were in financial difficulty.

Various small synagogues were also formed in Edinburgh. The most successful of these was for a time the shul in Richmond Street which served the Yiddish speaking immigrants. It was opened in 1895 and closed down in 1918. As time went on the Graham Street Synagogue expanded as the number of English speakers in the community increased. It was the local 'English' congregation where the more prosperous and assimilated members gathered. When Rabbi Salis Daiches arrived in Edinburgh in 1919 he received a call from both the Graham Street Synagogue and the members of the Roxburgh Place Beth Hamedrash, another small synagogue where Yiddish speakers and immigrants predominated.[43] Rabbi Daiches was initially held in a degree of suspicion by the Yiddish speakers who felt that he was too modern. Rabbi Daiches felt that the Graham Street Synagogue, while still Orthodox, 'clearly represented the wave of the future' as it had a higher proportion of Scottish born members.[44] In 1920 the two groups amalgamated and when the new synagogue was built in the Newington district they both came under the one roof.

During the 1920's there remained one dissident group known as the 'Bolshie Shul' who met in South Clerk Street. However, this group had the

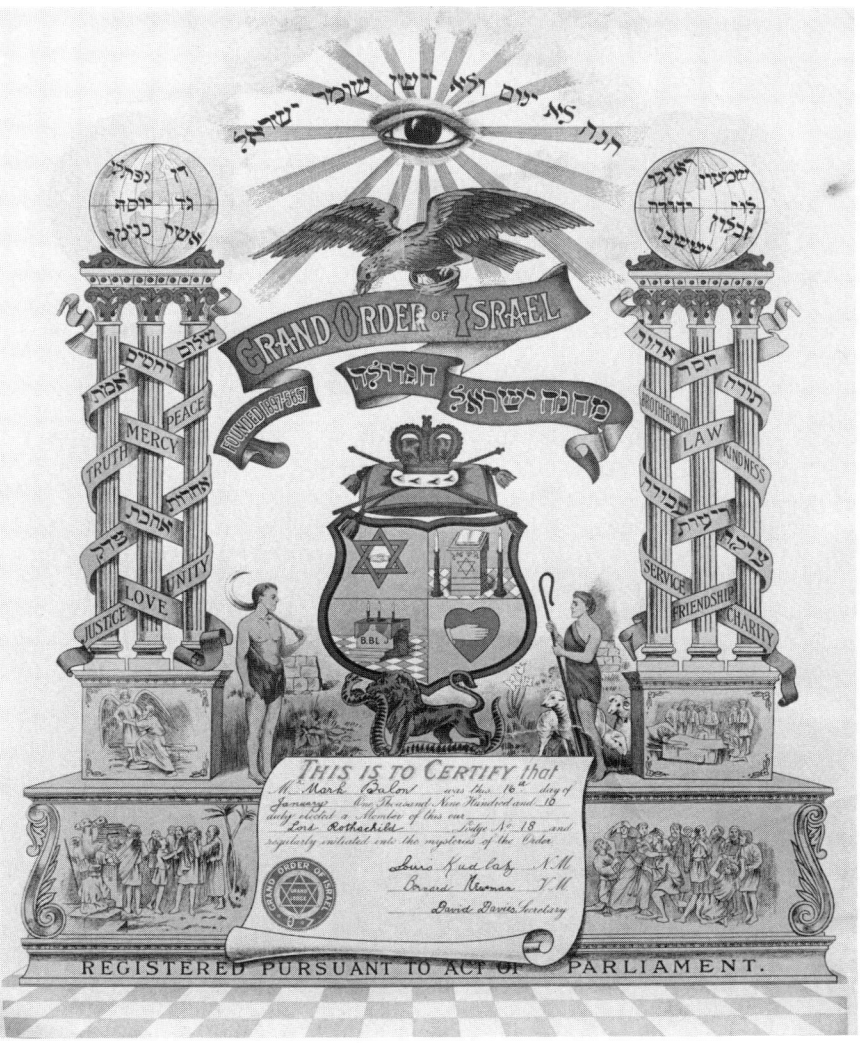

16 Membership certificate of one of the Jewish Friendly Societies in Glasgow, 1910
These societies provided much needed welfare and medical aid to the immigrants.

unfortunate experience of employing a minister who was the brother of two notorious missionaries and his forged credentials were exposed by Rabbi Daiches.[45,46] Eventually the two groups became reconciled to each other and communal unity in Edinburgh prevailed.

The religious patterns laid down by the 1930's set the trends for what was to follow later. The tenets of religious Orthodoxy observance which had come over with the immigrant generation, were followed to a lesser extent by their children. Laxity developed in the observance of the Sabbath, a trend accelerated by financial necessity at a time when the five day week was not yet the norm. Despite the flourishing network of Jewish foodstores it was clear that observance of the Jewish dietary laws was in decline especially outside the home. The laws of family purity were being ignored. Worse, there were allegations that it was money rather than 'personal piety and probity, religious spirit and intense Jewish consciousness' which characterised the synagogue lay leadership, who were, for the most part, unaware of the paradox of their behaviour.[47] Many of the practices and rituals of Orthodox Judaism call for a degree of continuing commitment which an increasing number found hard to follow.

Nevertheless, the drift from Orthodoxy was not accompanied by the rise of Reform Judaism in Scotland. Reform communities had been strongest in Britain where their tradition had been brought over from Germany, as in Bradford, or had been established earlier by more assimilated groups in London and Manchester. In this, the Glasgow pattern was closer to that of Leeds where the level of Orthodox affiliation remained high although there was a decline in its practice. There were none of the pressures to adapt Judaism to the norms of society as happened in America. In America the children of the immigrants often rebelled against the Orthodox synagogue practices typical of Eastern Europe forming Conservative synagogues which sought to preserve the important religious precepts while at the same time providing more decorous religious services. The integration of the children of the immigrants into Scottish society was accompanied by a certain distancing from the old ways. Children were often embarrassed by the alien ways and accents of their parents and were not afraid to express this publicly.[48] Nevertheless, these same children were content to remain within the framework of an Orthodoxy which preserved the old values but made little demands on its members and left the rabbinate isolated from the religiously lax behaviour of the new generation. The Orthodox synagogues in Scotland thus managed to accommodate a membership with a wide diversity of views, and a weakening attachment to religious practice. They appealed to the feeling that the synagogues were the main link with the Jewish traditions of 'der heim', and had to be preserved for that reason.

With the decline in religious observance it was not surprising that there were problems of intermarriage from the earliest years of the community and many of the families who arrived in Glasgow, Edinburgh and Dundee during the early and mid-nineteenth century gradually assimilated into their Scottish environment. There are no precise figures for intermarriage but there is a clear impression that this was on the rise during the 1920's and 1930's. It was said to be commoner for Jewish men marrying non-Jewish women to have their wives convert to Judaism than for Jewish women to have their non-Jewish husbands convert although examples of both can be found.[49] In particular, the Reform Synagogue in Glasgow came to boast a relatively high number of converts within its membership. Irregular acceptance of converts by various Jewish ministers, either acting as synagogue Rabbis or independently, was to cause much distress later on when the validity of such conversions was called into question. Many were found to be suspect. It is generally held that intermarriage was higher amongst the better educated groups, where access to higher education exposed them to the wider community, and among some of the poorer sections of the community whose level of attachment was less strong.[49]

Scottish Jewry did not always show great respect for its religious leadership and salaries were notoriously low. This in turn led to the need to augment income by means of teaching or accepting gratuities for the rendering of religious services. The lay leadership in the 1930's included many whose Jewish knowledge was hastily acquired and considerably forgotten in the struggle for economic survival. Thus while the Rabbi in Eastern Europe had been a figure inspiring great respect his standing in Scotland was somewhat lower.[50] The necessity to conform to the environment applied even to the Rabbis, as when Rabbi Azriel Bermant arrived in Glasgow in 1935 to take up the position of shochet he was taken aside by his colleagues and advised to trim his beard and remove the side-locks, which he used to have tucked behind his ears.[51]

If the religious leadership in Glasgow was passing to the Gorbals and South Side much of the secular leadership was still in the hands of the Garnethill and West End community. Glasgow had, in effect, two distinct Jewish communities until after the Second World War.[52] The Garnethill community stood for a more modern Orthodoxy, more worldly and more integrated with the non-Jewish society. Their ministers were Reverends rather than Rabbis and were products of Jews College and the universities rather than from the yeshiva world. The formation of volunteer groups and the founding of the Jewish Lads' Brigade, modelled on the Boys' Brigade, came from Garnethill.

Both Rabbi Daiches in Edinburgh and the Rev. Dr. I. K. Cosgrove, who came to Garnethill in 1935, had the aim of integrating the Jewish communities into the Scottish environment. They made close links with the wider national, civic and religious leadership and because of their high profile were widely referred to as the Chief Rabbis of Edinburgh and Glasgow. This aim of a synthesis of Scottish and Jewish culture was too elusive a goal for the Edinburgh community to follow but, as in Garnethill, there was a lively and informed Jewish community with an increasing professional and academic element which gradually paid less attention to the minutiae of Jewish observance. If Garnethill was the 'English' community of Glasgow then Edinburgh was an 'English' community, quiet, assimilated and increasingly well educated.

The Jews in Scotland tried to keep a low profile and always believed that any publicity was bad. When Rev. E. P. Phillips of Garnethill took up the case of Oscar Slater, a German Jew who had been wrongfully convicted of murder in Glasgow, it was made clear to him that he was acting independently of the synagogue.[53] There was always great care taken to ensure that community activities which of necessity took place on a Sunday were designed to cause as little offence as possible to Christian sensibilities.

The provision of Jewish education was one of the main communal priorities. It was motivated by the necessity of preserving as much as possible of traditional Jewish culture but quickly had to cope with the often conflicting needs of adapting to the educational needs which were necessary for eduational and social advancement in the wider society.

The first major Jewish educational institution in Glasgow, the Talmud Torah, was set up in 1895 in the Gorbals to provide elementary education and there were 400 pupils by 1899. Initially the language of instruction was Yiddish but this was changed to English before the First World War. This move was condemned by certain of the religious leaders as being assimilatory, and certainly it meant that the future of the Yiddish language was more precarious as its survival depended on its being learned in the home, where the pressures to speak English were all too obvious.

A framework of religious teaching followed the foundation of the new synagogues that developed both in the Gorbals and the new areas in which Jews were settling. The Talmud Torah contained the majority of pupils but many children were taught by individual teachers, known as melameds. These classes ran daily outwith school hours, usually meeting for a couple of hours at a time. Initially, the Talmud Torah classes met for three hours daily but the length of instruction was shortened, as an economy measure during the First World War and never increased again.[54] There was a considerable uptake of these facilities despite the pressures that the long hours of extra tuition must have placed on the Jewish pupils. They succeded because the priority of maintaining the Jewishness of the children of the immigrants was as strong as the pressure for the acculturation of their parents. Thus, whether it was in one of the chadarim in the Gorbals or in the basement of the Graham Street Synagogue in Edinburgh Jewish children were being instructed in the values which had motivated their parents in 'der heim'.

The idea of a Jewish day school was first mooted in Glasgow in 1910 and the Glasgow Jewish Representative Council took the matter up in 1914. They hoped to be able to take over one of the Gorbals schools as a Jewish school and indeed three of the primary schools in the Gorbals had 1,000 Jewish pupils, out of the total roll of 1,600. The Council's case was based on the long hours of study that Jewish pupils had to undertake which caused them to miss out on leisure time and interfered with homework.[55] In addition, it kept children from less committed homes from attending classes at all and some estimates of Jewish children missing out on Hebrew tuition were as high as 50%.

In 1920 the Glasgow Education Authority agreed to make over a school to the Jewish community as they accepted that the extra Jewish educational requirements were burdensome although they were worried that the move might prove to be divisive.[56] However, the insistence of limiting Jewish tuition

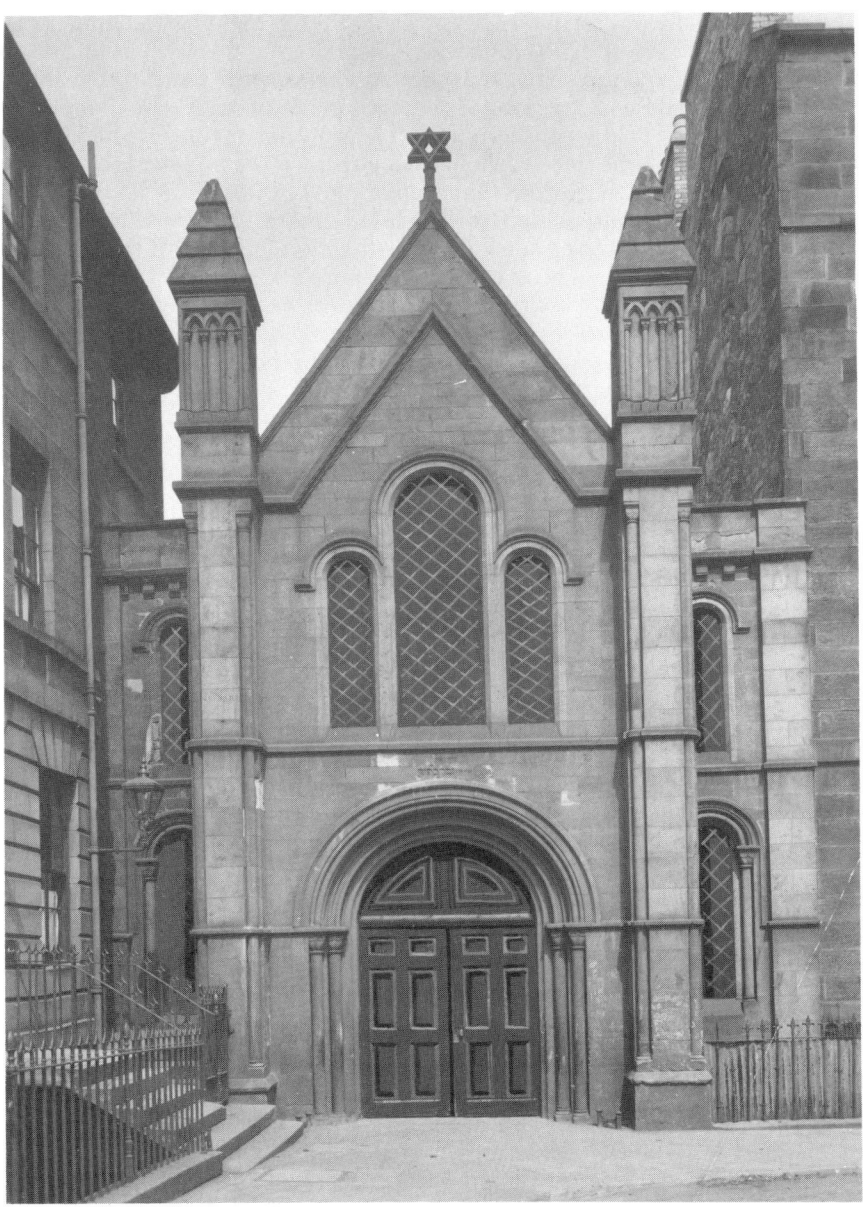

17 Graham Street Synagogue, Edinburgh, home of the Edinburgh Hebrew Congregation 1898–1932.

to one hour a day and the closing of the cheder network led to Jewish rejection of the proposal. By the 1920's the move out of the Gorbals was well underway although there were still 500 Jewish schoolchildren in the Gorbals in 1934.

The failure to establish a Jewish day school as the centre for the provision of Jewish studies caused increasing problems as time went on. As the community dispersed, mainly to the southern suburbs, problems increased. In 1916 it was estimated that one third of the Jewish girls received no Jewish education whatsoever [57] and twenty years later when only 1,000 out of 1,900 Jewish schoolchildren were attending Hebrew classes the situation was no better.[58] While the majority received some Jewish education for some of the time and there was a small group who managed to acquire a sound Hebrew education, all that could be achieved with the majority was basic Hebrew literacy and some familiarity with the main Jewish customs. These problems prompted the attempt to introduce some Hebrew studies into those schools where there was a considerable Jewish element, initially in the Gorbals and subsequently in Battlefield and Mount Florida. Again these attempts foundered as the period of time on offer at these schools was often less than an hour a day when many pupils were accustomed to attend Hebrew classes for upwards of ten hours weekly. There was a real fear that the provision of facilities for those who were obtaining none might be achieved at the expense of the larger number already within the Jewish educational system.

Many parents were worried about the idea of a Jewish school because, as immigrants or the children of immigrants, they still felt the need to be regarded as part of the wider community and did not wish to see their children segregated within the educational framework. They felt that the cheder system was adequate and that they could compensate for any deficiencies by the observance of Jewish customs at home. The religious establishment had a vested interest in maintaining the Jewish voluntary educational system which channelled the children of the community through their institutions. They were also apprehensive about the orientation of a Jewish day school where they might have little direct control. In fact a Jewish primary school was not established in Glasgow until 1962, still amidst opposition, when the battle for acceptance had been won and the danger to the community was perceived to be estrangement from Jewish culture and traditions.

Even in the inter-war period Jewish education was mainly aimed at the primary age group with very few secondary pupils obtaining any Jewish studies. This had been noted as early as 1903 and by the 1930's barely 10% of Jewish teenagers received any Jewish education whether in the Glasgow Yeshiva or in the Hebrew College, which offered a broad view of Hebrew and Jewish studies.[58]

In 1937 Glasgow possessed thirteen centres at which primary Jewish education was taught and it was acknowledged that the standards varied widely. Many of the teachers were graduates of the Hebrew College, often university students seeking to help to finance their studies and there were many medical students amongst them. As early as 1910 the majority of the teachers at the Garnethill Hebrew Classes were medical students[59] and indeed cheder teaching was once described as a form of undergraduate relief.[60]

Evening classes were provided at the Gorbals Public School from 1893 and these quickly expanded under the aegis of the Jewish Literary Society and H.M. Inspectorate.[61] However, Yiddish continued to be widely used in the community and at public meetings for many years.

There was a considerable network of informal Jewish education fostered by various youth groups and student and Young Zionist societies. Many of the synagogues possessed their own clubs and debating societies which catered for members of all ages. In 1928 the Zionist socialist pioneering youth movement Habonim was founded in Glasgow and twenty five years later it claimed to be the largest Jewish youth group in the city. Jewish sporting activities were fostered by the Jewish Institute, both in Glasgow and Edinburgh. The Glasgow Jewish Athletic Club was founded in 1921 and provided facilities for tennis and later for badminton also. The Bar Cochba Sports Club was formed in Glasgow in 1933 and quickly developed sections in all the major sports such as football, boxing and swimming and by 1937 it had 250 members.

Community awareness of the outside world was also enhanced by the activities of the local Jewish press. There had been a Yiddish paper *The Jewish Times* circulating in Glasgow around the turn of the century and in 1914 a Yiddish daily paper *The Glasgow Jewish Evening Times* was started but this soon became a weekly paper. During the 1920's Zevi Golombok, who had edited the *Glasgow Jewish Evening Times* founded a Yiddish language weekly called the *Jewish Voice* but owing to the falling numbers of Yiddish readers in

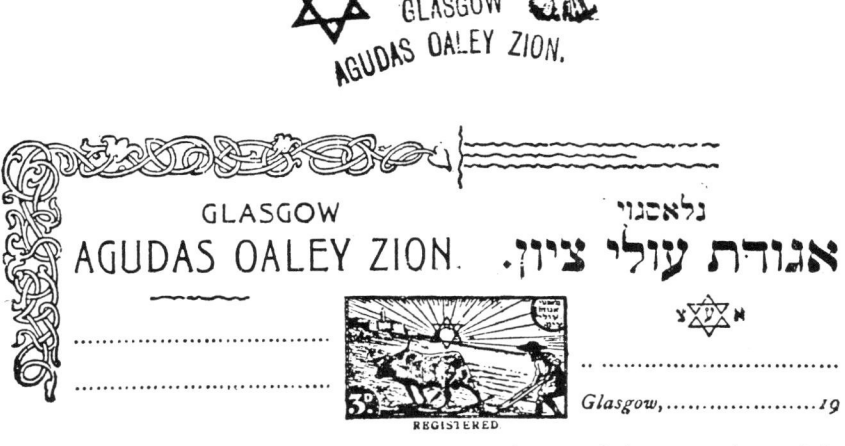

18   Glasgow Jewry's commitment to Zionism is long and deep. Members of the Agudas Oaley Zion settled in the Land of Israel before the Balfour Declaration.

the community he started an English language weekly Jewish newspaper in 1928 called the *Jewish Echo*. This paper was successful from the start and its columns provide an invaluable source of Jewish community history in Scotland. There were competitiors from time to time, such as the *Jewish Leader* during the 1930's but none survived long.

Golombok's concerns in the *Jewish Echo* for Zionism and Jewish rights in countries of oppression helped to shape popular opinion. The editor was not afraid to give his opinions on communal matters and the lively correspondence columns could often give clues to areas of communal concern.

By the 1930's therefore Scottish Jewry had become well established. Glasgow Jewry had increased in size from being one of the smallest Jewish communities in Britain only a century before, to become the third largest provincial community containing an estimated 15,000 Jews and being smaller only than Leeds (25,000) and Manchester (35,000).

There was an initial concern that the drift from the Gorbals would be associated with a break in community cohesion and that support for the Gorbals-based charities would be weakened.[62] This proved not to be the case as many in the more outlying areas depended on many of the facilities which were only available in the Gorbals. Some Jews who had dispersed to other parts of Glasgow where there was little Jewish life actually returned during this period to the Jewish warmth of the Gorbals. The Jewish community in Edinburgh had expanded to number about 2,500.

Jews were represented in the furniture and tailoring trades as well as in tobacco. A Jewish Tailors' Union was established in Glasgow in 1890 and a Jewish Workers' Union was set up in 1912. Sweat shop conditions were often appalling but much was tolerated in the drive to overcome the poverty of the early years. The Jewish self-employed were concentrated in hawking and peddling long after these activities had ceased to be standard Jewish occupations in London and Manchester. In 1906 it was estimated that there were 600 pedlars in Glasgow out of a community of about 8,000 while the percentage in Edinburgh was even higher.[63] Jews travelled from Glasgow to the mining villages of Ayrshire and Lanarkshire. From Edinburgh they travelled to Fife and from Falkirk round Stirlingshire. In Edinburgh, the pedlars or 'trebblers', developed their own Scots-Yiddish dialect.[64]

These trends were followed by the smaller Jewish communities in Scotland although communal activities were modified by the smaller scale. Depsite this a number of vibrant small Jewish groups existed for a time in various Scottish towns. Outside of Glasgow and Edinburgh the largest Jewish community was in Dundee where a number of German Jewish textile agents had settled. The community maintained a wide range of communal activities for the fifty Jewish families in the town with a synagogue in Meadow Street opened in 1919 and the services of a resident minister. In Aberdeen the Jewish community achieved national prominence shortly after its founding in 1893 when its minister and president were prosecuted by the local branch of the Society for the Prevention of Cruelty to Animals for its conduct of shechita. The case against the Aberdeen community was dismissed with the judgement accepting that the shechita had been conducted expertly.[65] By 1904 there

THE GROWTH AND DEVELOPMENT OF SCOTTISH JEWRY

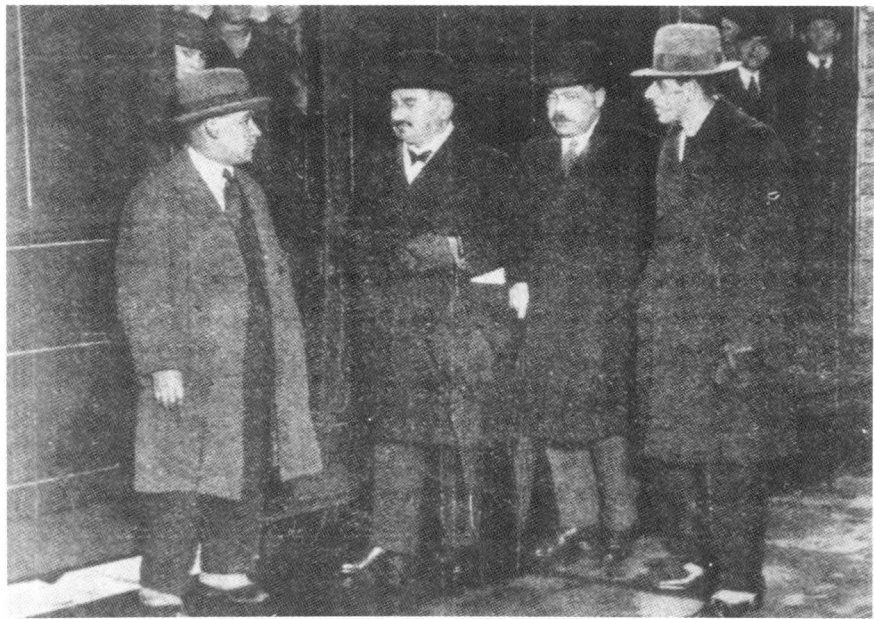

19   Rabbi Satis Daiches meets leaders of the Aberdeen Hebrew Congregation, 1926. Courtesy *Glasgow Herald*.

were seventeen Jewish families in Aberdeen but they continued to maintain level of communal activities which involved the members in considerable financial commitment.

Jews gathered in Greenock as a result of its position on the trans-shipment route and the first services there were held in 1894 and by 1920 there was a synagogue and a Jewish cemetery. However the community was dissolved by 1936 as the Jews began to leave town. The other small Jewish communities in Inverness, Ayr, Falkirk and Dunfermline grew as a result of internal immigration within Scotland with Jews looking for locations from which trade could be conducted with less competition than could be found in the larger centres. However, the viability of these small communities did not last for long, as their members tended to drift away to the larger centres of Jewish population in Glasgow and Edinburgh. Although there are still small Jewish communities today in Aberdeen and Dundee the story of Scottish Jewry has essentially been a 'tale of two cities'. Jews tended to move from the smaller centres especially as their children were growing up and they sought a wider social framework. Other Jews lived isolated from other Jews in towns and villages throughout Scotland from the Shetlands to the Borders. They were involved either in commercial activity, providing professional services or running the local store. Jewish contacts were maintained by links with Glasgow and Edinburgh and by the formation of a number of Scottish Jewish organisations, especially in the fields of welfare and education.

The occupational structure of the community had changed by the 1930's with more Jews entering various areas of remunerative employment and the formation of successful businesses. Some Jews were still to be found in peddling but many more were to be found in the traditional activities of clothing, shopkeeping and furniture. Although most Jews worked outside the slump-ridden heavy engineering sector, studies showed that Jewish receipt of welfare was higher than for their non-Jewish neighbours.[66] At Passover in 1937 no fewer than 1,400 Glasgow Jews were in receipt of relief from the Glasgow Jewish Board of Guardians, a figure approaching 10% of the community.[67] Yet while there was still widespread poverty within the community, as there was outside it, in economic terms tremendous strides had been made during the previous thirty years. While a large Jewish labour market persisted, the second and third generation of Jews settled in Glasgow and Edinburgh were moving increasingly into their own businesses, into the professions, white collar jobs and generally into wider areas of employment.

By the 1930's there was a clear trend of movement into the professions in Scottish Jewry represented mainly by an increasing number entering medicine. Jews did not find it easy to enter the conservative Scottish law firms and 70% of Jewish undergraduates in Glasgow in 1936 gave medicine as their first career choice.[68] Only medicine was seen as a passport to a clearly defined career and parents were willing to make the necessary financial sacrifices for their sons to enter the medical profession.

Jewish student activities at the Universities of Edinburgh and Glasgow began with the informal gathering together of Jewish students to discuss contemporary Zionist issues. In Edinburgh, the University Jewish Society was founded in 1909 after some debate about the advisability of such a move.[69] Some Jewish students were concerned that a Jewish Society might be divisive and separate the Jewish students from other groups on campus. The majority of Jewish students in Edinburgh were from overseas and especially from South Africa. The Chief Rabbi had met a group of Jewish students 'from the Empire' during his visit to Edinburgh in 1907.[68] Zionist activity on campus was promoted from 1909 by Lewis Rifkind who later qualified as a doctor and was also a spokesman for the socialist Poalei Zion Party.[70]

Following the First World War the Jewish Society at Edinburgh University re-formed and the increased numbers of local Jews entering university balanced the fall in the number of South African Jews coming to study. However, the South African influence in the University Jewish Society continued until the 1930's. By this time substantial numbers of American Jews were arriving in Edinburgh to study medicine although they were organised in the American Medical Club and only a few were active in the Jewish Students' Society.

Although the Jewish Students' Society was not formed in Glasgow until January 1912, fully two years after its counterpart in Edinburgh, there had already been some organised Jewish undergraduate activity in the city.[71] The Glasgow Young Men's Zionist Cultural Assocation had been found in 1908 with a mainly undergraduate membership. By 1911 the dozen Jewish students at Gilmorehill, most of whom were studying medicine, were mindful of developments in Zionism and the persecutions of the Jews in Russia and Rumania as well as participating in the wider student issues of the day. They felt that it was important that Jewish students organise together for the discussion of Jewish topics and affairs. One of the original aims of those founding the Jewish Students' Society was the strengthening of Jewish identity both on campus and after graduation.

The Jewish Students' Society was not formed in Glasgow without some discussion, as there had been in Edinburgh, about the propriety of such a move.[71] Some Jewish students felt that such a group would not be welcome by the university authorities and others thought that the mere organising together of Jewish students would be inviting anti-semitism. There was also a fear that the students' strong affiliation to political Zionism, which was warmly endorsed by the mainstream of Gorbals Jewry, would be less sympathetically received by the more assimilated Jewish leaders of the day. Despite the objections an enthusiastic majority agreed to organise the Glasgow University Jewish Society with Samuel Grasse as its first President and the Professor of Hebrew, W. B. Stevenson, was elected Honorary President and delivered the inaugural lecture.

Thus by the outbreak of the Second World War the condition of Scottish Jewry had been transformed. There was considerable social, educational and economic advance and there was little serious anti-semitism even in the Gorbals where the Jews had formed a significant and visible minority. The challenge facing Jews in Scotland was to survive as Jews outside the 'ghetto' areas. This was achieved by the the founding of new organisations which replaced the original groups set up by the newcomers. As religious groups weakened it was necessary to form more social societies to preserve the links between the members of the community. Marrying out of the faith was considered to be a disgrace for the whole family and it was important to find ways of fostering a community spirit. Scottish Jewry thus continued as a cohesive society despite the weakening of religious links and the gradual disappearance of the Yiddish language, which had not proved to be an essential element in preserving Jewish identity.

Communal cohesion had been strengthened by the response to missionary activities. Many of the more innovative welfare campaigns followed attempts by the missionaries to attract impoverished or lonely Jews by offering them facilities not available within the Jewish community. Glasgow Jewry, and also Edinburgh Jewry, responded to these moves by founding societies and providing welfare schemes which were freely admitted to be related to thwarting missionary success.[72] Scottish Jewry was considerably stronger as a result.

By the 1930's the integration of Scottish Jewry was gaining momentum. Scottish Jews had become an established part of the Scottish scene with many achievements in many aspects of community, national and political life.

Within the Jewish community upward social mobility was fostered by the desire of the communal elite to assimilate the community to British middle class norms and to provide for a rapid 'Anglicisation' of the Jewish immigrants. Thus the early years of the community saw the establishment of classes in the English language and more significantly the formation of volunteer groups to stress Jewish loyalty to the new country. A large, though often underfunded, communal welfare network ensured that immigrant Jews would not be a charge on the host community. The emergence, after the Second World War, of two occupational groupings in Anglo-Jewry, namely business or mercantile and professional, can be traced back to the early years of the community when the career options of the children of the immigrants was to break away from the ghetto trades or to enter the burgeoning businesses started by their fathers.

The priorities of the first generation had been the establishment of an economic base, thereby creating the conditions which would enable their children to reap the rewards to which the parents could not aspire. With a protectively warm and secure family life, and the ethos which gave religious and secular education a high priority, the new generation gradually moved out of the world of the petty trader, artisan and pedlar into one where success would be measured by academic achievement.

REFERENCES

1 A.Levy, *The Origins of Scottish Jewry*, Paper read to the JHSE on 13 Jan. 1958, p.8
2 *Jewish Encyclopaedia*, (New York 1925) Vol.X1 pp.424-5
3 David Daiches, *Glasgow*, (1977) p.136
4 Charles J. Withers, 'Kirk, Club and Culture change: Gaelic chapels, Highland Societies and the urban Gaelic sub-culture in eighteenth century Scotland' *Social History*, (1985) Vol.10 no.2, pp.171-92
5 *Jewish Chronicle* 19 Aug. 1881
6 Bill Williams, *The Making of Manchester Jewry 1740-1875* (Manchester, paperback reprint, 1985) p.328
7 Chaim Bermant, *Troubled Eden*, (1969) p.221
8 *Encyclopaedia Judaica*, (Jerusalem, 1972) Vol.15, col.1042
9 C. C. Aronsfeld, 'German Jews in Dundee', *Jewish Chronicle* 20 Nov. 1953
10 Chaim Bermant op.cit., pp.25-7
11 *Jewish Chronicle* 15 Dec. 1905
12 *Jewish Chronicle* 6 Feb. 1903
13 Rayner Kolmel, 'Problems of Settlement : German Jewish Refugees in Scotland', *Exile in Great Britain: Refugees from Hitler's Germany*, Gerhard Hirschfeld (ed.), (New Jersey 1984) pp.258, 266-70
14 A. Levy, 'The Early Days of Glasgow Jewry', *Hashanah 1955-1956*, (Glasgow 1955) p.45
15 *Jewish Chronicle* 8 Mar. 1878
16 A. Levy, *The Origins of Scottish Jewry*, p.18
17 Personal interviews, S.L, A.R.
18 Jack Ronder, *The Lost Tribe* (1978) pp.22-30
19 Lloyd P. Gartner, *The Jewish Immigrant in England 1870-1914* (1973) p.74
20 *Jewish Year Book* 1896

21 *Jewish Chronicle* 13 Sept. 1901
22 *Jewish Chronicle* 26 Nov. 1886
23 *Jewish Chronicle* 2 June 1905
24 *Jewish Chronicle* 30 Dec. 1910
25 *Glasgow Jewish Year Book* 1937, p.23
26 ibid., p.55
27 *Jewish Chronicle* 7 June 1889
28 *Jewish Chronicle* 17 and 24 Feb. 1911
29 'Profile of Bernard Glasser at 85', *Jewish Echo*, 20 Sept. 1957
30 *Glasgow Herald* 23 Nov. 1906
31 *Jewish Chronicle* 31 Aug. 1919
32 *Jewish Chronicle* 12 May 1922
33 *Jewish Chronicle* 6 Mar. 1925
34 *Jewish Chronicle* 9 Nov. 1934
35 *Jewish Chronicle* 22 Feb. 1929
36 *Jewish Chronicle* 28 May 1897
37 *Jewish Chronicle* 14 Feb. 1902
38 Chaim Bermant, *Coming Home* (1976) p.37
39 Montague Jacobs, 'Our Community and its Institutions', *Glasgow Jewish Year Book* 1937, p.39
40 *Jewish Chronicle* 18 Feb. 1921
41 *Glasgow Herald* 11 Oct. 1913
42 *Jewish Chronicle* 18 Oct. 1901
43 David Daiches, *Two Worlds* (Sussex 1957) p.98
44 ibid., p.97
45 ibid., pp.100-104
46 Jewish Chronicle 2 June 1922, 21 Dec. 1923, 7 Nov. 1924
47 *Lewis Rifkind* (Glasgow n.d.)
48 *Jewish Chronicle* 26 Jan. 1923
49 Personal interviews, on file
50 Chaim Bermant op.cit., p.39
51 Chaim Bermant op.cit., p.37
52 Chaim Bermant, 'Anatomy of Glasgow', in B. Mindlin and C. Bermant (eds.) *Explorations* (1967) p.103
53 Minute Book of the Garnethill Hebrew Congregation 16 Sept. 1909
54 'Some Happy Reminiscences of an Old Talmud Torah Pupil' *Glasgow Hebrew College Magazine*, p.7-9
55 *Glasgow Chronicle* 19 June 1914
56 *Glasgow Herald* 7 May 1920
57 *Jewish Chronicle* 16 June 1916
58 Dr. M. Friedlander, 'Glasgow Jewish Education: A Survey of Activities' *Glasgow Jewish Year Book* 1937, p.25
59 Garnethill Hebrew Congregation, *Annual Report of School Committee* 1909-1910
60 Chaim Bermant, *Troubled Eden* (1969) p.57
61 *Jewish Chronicle* 23 Oct. 1896
62 *Jewish Echo* 11 Sept. 1936
63 Lloyd P. Gartner ibid., p.60
64 David Daiches op.cit., p.119
65 *Glasgow Jewish Year Book* 1937, p.23
66 *Jewish Chronicle* 7 Sept. 1903
67 Geoffrey D. Block and Harry Schwab, 'Jewish Students: A Survey of their Position at the Universities of Great Britain'. *Jewish Year Book* 1938, p.372

68 *Jewish Chronicle* 8 Jan. 1909 and 15 Jan. 1909
69 *Jewish Chronicle* 14 June 1907
70 *Jewish Echo* 1 July 1937
71 *Jewish Echo* 1 Mar. 1961
72 *Jewish Chronicle* 31 July 1914

FIVE

The Movement of Jews into the Medical Profession in Scotland from 1880

Although the Jewish population was very small in Scotland during the nineteenth century, there were signs of an interest in the professions from an early period. By 1859 there had been five Scots Jewish medical graduates from the Scottish universities at a time when there were less than 500 Jews in all Scotland. That there were few Scottish Jews entering medicine in Edinburgh and Glasgow in the last decades of the nineteenth century can be attributed both to the small size and poverty of the community and to the financial rewards which could be obtained in business and commerce, especially in the 'Second City' of the Empire. Nonetheless, the fact that Samuel Levenston twice acted as trustee for the Glasgow Hebrew Congregation, the first time while still a medical student, suggests the respect in which professional learning was held.

For the first generation of immigrants the overwhelming priority was economic survival. This involved work in a variety of craft and labouring occupations and in the sweated workshops of the garment trade as well as in hawking and peddling. Despite the formation of large Jewish groups in working class occupations in some of the great urban centres of Britain and America, Jewish parental attitudes fitted closely into the middle class attitudes of 'getting on' and of a man being judged by what he makes of himself.[1] Jewish experience also showed that setting up in business did not act as a bar to the pursuit of middle class values among the working class. In addition, while parental expectation among the non Jewish working classes was high, their desire that these hopes will be translated into real career chances for their children was weak.[1] Again, this does not correlate with the Jewish experience

While the immigrant generation might succeed in working themselves up a little they were still caught in the grip of the old ways.[2] They were trapped by the limitation of their skills and the awkwardness of their English, the skimpiness of their formal education and their alien manners. It was their sons who would achieve collective Jewish fulfilment and individual Jewish success. It does not matter that the immigrants themselves would have found this a difficult concept to grasp, they simply lived it out in their own experiences, coming to understand later what had happened.

Orthodox immigrants feared for the weakening of their faith on the pathway to emancipation and assimilation.[3] Socialist Jews shunned material fulfilment which might render utopian goals irrelevant. Yet for the vast bulk of the newcomers the question was the matter of economic necessity and survival.

At first many found occupations within the framework of the community but for most it was essential to survive in the outside world. This involved the acquisition of language skills and included an early movement into clerical work and into the professions.

Jews began to move into medicine in Scotland within a few years of the start of the large scale immigration. It took a number of years for a group of children who had been educated in English to develop but there were cases of students, such as Meyer Mann (Teitelmann), son of the Edinburgh cantor, entering university after only a year or two at a Scottish secondary school. The majority of the Scottish Jewish students at university before the First World War were studying medicine and this continued unchanged as the numbers of students increased substantially over the following decades

Scottish medicine was receptive to the newcomers. There was a significant working class element who saw in medicine the road to social advancement,[4] [5] in keeping with the Scottish tradition of the democratic ideal in education. The idea that social advancement through medical qualification came about through individual ambition and collective effort applies as much to the generality of doctors as it does to Jewish doctors from immigrant families. The transformation of medicine, with the aid of numerous advances in medical science, led to a greater expectation of success. Doctors were able to assume greater authority in their dealings with their patients and they realised the social value which was being placed on their work. Conditions were being set for the upward mobility of general practitioners within the medical profession despite the control over the profession wielded by an elite determined to maintain their own social status.[6]

The status of the medical profession in Glasgow rose steadily in the last decades of the nineteenth century as a reflection of the city's burgeoning prosperity.[7] The increased number of skilled workers created a more dependable demand for medical care which brought improvements even to those in the lower ranks of the profession. With the development of insurance society work practitioners could exchange a degree of professional freedom for a degree of security, in the form of State intervention.[8] Thus the medical profession was increasingly regarded as a more desirable occupation.

Possibilities existed for medical studies to be conducted economically. Although many doctors were trapped in activities which carried a low salary there were compensations such as security of employment and the chance of utilisation of the contacts made, such as on management committees, to further career prospects.[9] Hospital boards of management were increasingly attracted by the aura of success and wished to employ the best medical talent available. Nepotism and the existence of close religious or ethnic ties between doctor and patient did not disappear but there was scope for the development of achievement on merit. It is true that the majority of recruits into Scottish medicine came from the children of the middle class but there was still room for the Scottish 'lad o' pairts' and the Jewish immigrant tailor's son. The traditional absence of religious tests for entry into university also helped in the development of the early Jewish professional community.

The conditions were thus favourable for the entry of Scottish Jews into the medical profession. The goal increasingly became a place at the medical schools in Edinburgh and Glasgow as studying at home carried financial advantages. It was cheaper to live at home and there were opportunities to supplement income by additional work in such areas as tutoring. Few of the students had private means and the majority of Jewish students in Scotland relied on scholarships to help fund their undergraduate studies.[10] It was the Carnegie Trust for the Universities of Scotland, which from 1901 disbursed an annual income of £100,000, which provided the funds which made it possible for those who needed financial assistance for their studies to enter universities. It may not have transformed the conditions of access as Carnegie's critics said, but its contribution was hardly negligible.[11] This was especially true for the Jewish students who, as we shall see, had a high take up of Carnegie awards

While Jews took up available scholarship funds, such as those provided by the Carnegie Trust, there was a fund set up at St. Andrews University with the specific aim of supporting two Jewish students there.[12] This fund was established by the Marquess of Bute, who was Rector of the University of St. Andrews from 1892 to 1898, and administered through the Office of the Chief Rabbi in London. The scholarship was awarded regularly until the early 1970's when it was thought that its restrictive character might offend against race relations legislation. As medical students formed the majority of Jewish students at St. Andrews in the interwar years it is likely that a regular number of Jewish medical students benefitted from the Bute award. The financial dependence underlined the need to enter a career where there were prospects of material, as well as social, advance.

By the beginning of the First World War about twenty Scottish Jews had graduated in medicine and amongst these were the founders of the Jewish student societies in Glasgow and Edinburgh. The rapid growth in the number of Jews entering medicine continued in the years after the War. From 18 between 1910 and 1919 the numbers increased to 32 between 1920 and 1924 and to 51 between 1925 and 1929. There were many factors involved. There was the tradition of respect which Jews had for medicine and the physician, and for the scientific and secular learning that being a doctor implied. The doctor was seen as a figure of respect, not only within the immigrant world but within the wider Scottish society. In addition, possession of a medical qualification was seen as a prime asset in a community only recently established after much hardship in a strange land. The strong Jewish sense of pride in the achievements of children and the willingness to make economic sacrifices were also of crucial importance. Medicine was seen as the main professional target for Jewish students from the earliest days of Jewish entry to the universities. Although there were a few arts and law students amongst the first group of organised Jewish students in Glasgow, the majority were medical. The Scottish legal profession was perceived as being difficult to penetrate and partnerships in the conservative law firms were hard to obtain.[13] In addition, a qualification in Scots law meant a limited geographical choice in the place of the graduate's future career. In England the percentage of Jewish students entering law was 8% of the Jewish student body, the same percentage as in Glasgow. By contrast, there was only one Jewish law student in Edinburgh in 1936-7.[14]

The Jewish entry into medicine in Scotland was impressive even in comparison with trends in other western countries to which Jewish emigrants had been attracted. Within one generation of the arrival of groups of destitute Jewish refugees in Scotland, with no knowledge of the English language or the mores of Scottish society, and with their Jewish ways as their common identity, a considerable professional element had emerged (Table 5:1).

Jews were entering medicine throughout Europe, as well as in North America and South America. By 1925 Jews had formed more than 10% of the medical profession in Prussia, Hungary and the Soviet Union.[15] In South Africa, as we have seen, the figure was even higher. In many parts of urban Central Europe Jews formed large minorities while in Scotland the Jewish community never exceeded half of one per cent of the population.

The movement of Jews into medicine in Scotland did not occur without some degree of prejudice or anti-semitism, although such charges are always hard to substantiate. There was, for example, a continuing suspicion amongst Jewish graduates in Glasgow that it was particularly difficult for Jews to obtain house officer posts in Glasgow's main teaching hospitals, the Royal and Western Infirmaries.[16] In the early years of the century a few Jews had obtained posts there. Palestine born Reuben Youdelevitz-Young was appointed house officer at the Glasgow Royal Infirmary in 1906 only a year after Simon Sperber, of Montreal, had become the first Jew to be appointed to the staff of the Edinburgh Royal Infirmary and a few others held similar posts in the following years.

However, despite the great increase in the numbers of Jewish medical graduates during the 1920's and 1930's there was no corresponding increase in the number of Jewish house officers in the major Glasgow teaching hospitals.[17] At the Western Infirmary, for example, there were no Jewish house officers between 1921 and 1941, out of over 700 appointments, although there were a couple during the Second World War. At the Glasgow Royal Infirmary there were two Jewish house officers, out of over 300, during the 1930's.

Table 5:1   Scottish Jews entering medicine 1900-1945

Triple Qualif	LRCP&SE, LRFPS	Univ. of Glasgow	Univ. of Edinburgh	Univ. of Aberdeen	Univ. of St. Andrews	Total
1900-9	-	-	1	-	-	1
1910-4	-	7	3	-	-	10
1915-9	2	4	2	-	-	8
1920-4	9	17	4	-	2	32
1925-9	13	28	9	-	1	51
1930-4	10	28	5	-	-	43
1935-9	30	40	12	1	1	84
1940-5	44	33	11	-	-	88

(Extracted from graduation albums, 1900-1945)

During the First World War there had been accusations that Jewish doctors, in areas with a high proportion of immigrant Jews, were giving medical exemptions from military service in cases which were not justifiable on medical grounds.[18] Naturally, immigrant Jews were not keen to fight for the allies of the Russian Tsar, but such accusations cannot be found in the records of the Ministry of National Service concerning other groups in society. These allegations parallelled suggestions in Glasgow that immigrant Jews were trying to avoid the draft.[19]

Most Jews saw their advancement in medicine as a means of economic and social progress while retaining active membership of the Jewish community. For others the medical degree was the passport out of the community. Alfred Finkelstein, who had graduated at the University of Glasgow in 1895 and was the first Jew to serve as Medical Officer to the Glasgow Jewish Board of Guardians, later ceased to identify with the community.[20]

The Scottish medical schools produced more doctors than Scotland's population required and there was always a regular medical emigration. The Jewish doctors qualifying in Scotland merely followed this trend, either settling in England or even going overseas. Louis Turiansky who graduated in Edinburgh in 1903 and had been noted as a student of the Talmud during his student days, settled in London. He practised at 10 Osborn Street in the East End, acted as doctor to the residents of the Rothschild Buildings and was a conspicuous figure with his top hat and pony and trap.[21] Hyam Goodman, a former pupil of Hutcheson's Grammar School in Glasgow and the first Jewish President of the Students' Representative Council of Glasgow University, graduated in 1899 and later settled in Johannesburg.[22]

There were only four Jewish doctors practising in Glasgow on the eve of the First World War. These included Saul Harris who qualified in 1910 and was for many years the senior Jewish medical figure in the city. He had been the first Medical Officer of the Jewish Dispensary, which had been opened in 1911 by the Glasgow Jewish Board of Guardians, to serve the poor Jews in Gorbals who were being enticed to the Medical Halls of the numerous active Christian missionary groups.[23] Another was Meyer Mann, who had qualified in Edinburgh in 1913, and was for many years the Medical Officer of the Gertrude Jacobson Orphanage for Jewish children. Simon Harry Bennett gained his M.B. Ch.B in 1913 and proceeded M.D. in 1917 for his work on the complications of trauma and neurasthenia. He served as extra dispensing physician at the Glasgow Royal Infirmary. The fourth was Noah Morris who had a distinguished medical career culminating in his being appointed to the Regius Chair of Materia Medica at the University of Glasgow in 1937.

Morris had proceeded M.D. with honours in 1921 and was awarded the Bellahouston Gold Medal. In 1920 he was appointed Professor of Physiology at Anderson's College, one of the Glasgow extra-mural medical schools, a post he held for eight years. When he was appointed to the Regius Chair in 1937 a dinner was organised under the auspices of the Garnethill Synagogue as it was widely felt that this honour marked a further step in the integration of the Jewish community into the life of the city.[24] In fact, the community took particular pride in this appointment as Morris symbolised the successful combination of the Jewish scholar who was equally at home in the wider world. Morris had been the founder, lecturer and Chairman of the Glasgow Hebrew college, was an active member of the Glasgow Board of Jewish Education and was Chairman of the Glasgow Friends of the Hebrew University of Jerusalem.

During the 1920's more Jews began to enter university, mostly to study medicine. In the 1920's there would not have been more than two dozen Jewish medical students at Glasgow University at any one time but their number steadily expanded during the 1930's Medicine was the subject chosen overwhelmingly by Jewish students in Scotland in the interwar period. In 1935, out of the 63 Jewish students recorded in the Glasgow *Jewish Echo* as having obtained passes in their undergraduate studies, no less than 43 did so in medicine.[25] A survey of Jewish students in Britain, between 1936 and 1939, showed that the preponderance of Jewish students in medicine, at 73%, was higher in Glasgow than in any other centre.[26] This concentration in medicine was receiving attention within the Glasgow Jewish community. At a meeting of the Glasgow Junior Zionist Society in September, 1935 Dr. Meyer T. Mann said that he could not understand why anti-semitism was so rife in medicine. He said that it was extremely difficult for Jews to obtain hospital posts and he advised the Jewish youth of Glasgow to seek employment elsewhere as the medical profession was already filled to overflowing.[27]

The interwar period marked the shift of the Eastern European immigrants, and their children, into the professions. In the economic sphere Jewish businesses were prospering though confined to certain narrow sectors like textiles, retailing and furniture. Jews were also entering higher education, especially at the universities, in greater numbers. Nationally, as in Glasgow, medicine was the most popular professional career choice throughout the 1930's.[28] It had the advantage of the certainty of post-graduate employment and it carried a higher status within the immigrant community than did teaching. In fact, in traditional Jewish society, the high general level of Hebrew literacy ensured a continuing lowly status for the melamed, the teacher of basic Jewish studies.

There was some graduate unemployment during the 1930's especially in teaching[26] and this gave further impetus to the move into medicine as did parental expectation and economic necessity. Between 1934 and 1939 Jewish medical graduates in Scotland totalled 84 and the numbers increased again in the next 5 year period. Not all the students who started medical courses managed to complete their studies and not all those who qualified as doctors practised their professions. There are examples of Jewish doctors in both Edinburgh and Glasgow who entered the family businesses, whether clothing, furniture or electrical.[29]

Jewish women were studying at university, in small numbers, from the beginning of the twentieth century. Their numbers increased slowly during the 1920's and 1930's but did not rise significantly until the 1940's. At the University of Glasgow women made up 22% of the student body but only 10% of the Jewish students were women.[30] Jewish parents were protective towards their daughters and sought to keep them from university influences, and the contacts they might meet there. There was also the worry that long

Table 5:2 Estimated Jewish Population in Scotland 1935-1939

Glasgow	15,000
Edinburgh	2,500
Dundee	150
Aberdeen	150
Dunfermline	50
Falkirk	50
Inverness	50

source : Jewish Year Books

years spent in studies would make their daughters unmarriageable, a serious concern in a community where family life was so pivotal. The first Jewish woman to graduate in medicine in Scotland was Vera Dagmar Reis, who qualified at the University of Glasgow in 1906 but there were few others before the 1920's.[31]

Outside the major Scottish Jewish communities of Edinburgh and Glasgow there were only a few hundred Jews scattered around the country from Inverness and Aberdeen in the north, to Dumfries in the south (Table 5:2).

Even from such small Jewish communities as Aberdeen, Inverness, Falkirk and Dundee, there were a few medical graduates. Almost all left these Scottish towns and cities and the contribution of Dr. David Jacob, who graduated at St.Andrews in 1922, and remained active in the Dundee Jewish community, was unique in this respect (Table 5:3).

This entry of Jews into medicine in all the medical schools in Scotland led to a Jewish level of qualifications in medicine fully ten times their proportion in the general population.

At the University of Glasgow, Jewish medical graduates made up between 3.5% and 5.42% of the total between 1925 and 1945, although Jews formed less than 1% of the population of the university's catchment area in the West

Table 5:3 Scottish Jews entering medicine 1900-1945 by place of residence

| | Glasgow | | Edinburgh | | Others | | Total | |
	Triple	Univ.	Triple	Univ.	Triple	Univ.	Triple	Univ.
1900-9	-	-	-	1	-	-	-	1
1910-4	-	7	-	3	-	-	-	10
1915-9	1	4	1	2	-	-	2	6
1920-4	5	17	4	4	-	2	9	23
1925-9	6	28	6	9	1	1	13	38
1930-4	6	28	4	5	-	-	10	33
1935-9	26	40	3	12	1	2	30	54
1940-5	31	33	13	11	-	-	44	44

(Extracted from graduation albums, 1900-1945)

Table 5:4 Scottish Jewish Students Qualifying in Medicine

	Edinburgh Univ.		Glasgow Univ.		Triple qualification	
	no.	% of all medical graduates	no.	% of all medical graduates	no.	% of all medical graduates
1915-19	2		4		2	
1920-24	4	0.33	17	1.75	9	2.17
1925-29	9	1.31	28	3.50	13	2.03
1930-34	5	0.70	28	4.04	10	1.71
1935-39	12	1.52	40	5.42	30	5.23
1940-45	11	1.27	33	4.00	44	7.13

note: figures exclude Germans and Americans (745 between 1930 & 1945)
source: graduation albums of the Universities and the Triple Qualification Board

of Scotland. Glasgow Jews who took the Triple Qualification between 1935 and 1945 also formed between 4 and 5% of those qualifying.

In the smaller Jewish community in Edinburgh, similar trends were evident. Jews made up less than half of one per cent of the population of the city of Edinburgh. By 1925 their proportion among university medical graduates exceeded 1% and the proportion qualifying at university or in the extra-mural medical schools increased steadily during the next two decades (Table 5:4).

In the five years between 1935 and 1939 no less than 14% of the cohort group of Glasgow Jewish males, aged between 19 and 24 years, qualified in medicine and the Edinburgh figure was even higher at 20% (Table 5:5).

Even when the universities in Scotland began to limit the numbers of overseas students studying, many of whom were Jewish, there was never any evidence produced that local Jewish students with the right entry qualifications were being excluded.[32] In fact, the large number of medical places available in Scotland, and the policy of reserving places for local students, meant that there were places for any Scot who could meet the entry requirements. Indeed, during the early 1930's the universities were prepared to admit more local students had there been more available with the right qualifications. Thus Scotland was one of the few centres, with Dublin possibly another, where there were enough medical school places for any native Jew who wished to avail himself of one during the period.

During the 1930's there were more British Jews studying medicine in

Table 5:5

	Glasgow	Edinburgh
Size of 1935-1939 cohort group	950	150
Scottish Jewish qualifications in medicine	66	15
% of total	6.95%	10%
% of males in group	13.68%	20%

Glasgow than in any other British centre outside London, and that included Manchester and Leeds where the Jewish communities were larger than in Glasgow. Even more remarkably, the numbers in Edinburgh of local Jews studying medicine was not far behind those in the major English cities.[33] As the 1930's progressed the numbers of Jews entering the extra-mural medical schools in Glasgow and Edinburgh rose sharply. By 1940-1945 they outnumbered the Jews studying medicine in the universities, who had made up three quarters of the total only ten years before (Table 5:6).

Economic factors must have played a part in this. Fees at the extra-mural colleges were lower than at the universities and entry qualifications, while similar, could be applied more flexibly. With no less than 80 out of 102 Jewish students in Glasgow in 1938-9 in receipt of scholarships, the financial arguments seem important.[34] In Edinburgh 12 out of 17 local students were receiving scholarships compared with a minority of non-Jewish students. That the level of Jewish students in Scotland was higher than their co-religionists in other British cities may be attributed to the existance of Carnegie grants and was also an indication that a higher proportion of Scottish Jews were entering university. At a time when the number of Jews permitted to enter medicine was falling in Europe, because of discrimination and persecution, and in America because of implementation of a Jewish quota, the proportion of Jews entering medicine in Scotland was reaching a peak.

With the Scottish medical schools producing only one third less medical graduates than the English medical schools, it was inevitable that a large proportion of the Scottish doctors would follow the trend of leaving home in search of employment. During the 1920's less than half of the Jewish medical graduates from the University of Glasgow remained in Scotland, mostly in the Glasgow area itself.[35] There was a preponderance of general practitioners but a number of distinguished consultants emerged. During the 1930's as the numbers of Jews entering medicine increased substantially, less than one third of Jewish doctors remained in Scotland.

The Glasgow Jewish medical students came from a wide variety of backgrounds. As the professional element in the community was small, students who had professional fathers formed the smallest group, being mostly the sons of the rabbis, cantors and ministers of the various Glasgow synagogues. This group formed a greater proportion of the total before 1925. The remain-

Table 5:6 Jews qualifying in medicine in Glasgow

	Extra-mural	University	% extra-mural
1910-9	1	11	8.3
1920-9	11	45	19.6
1930-4	6	28	17.6
1935-9	26	40	39.4
1940-5	31	33	48.4

source: University and Triple Qualification Board Graduation Albums.

der were fairly evenly divided into the entrepreneurial category (those who owned or managed large businesses), the small business, artisan and the clerical and agents group (this last category included commercial travellers and two pedlars). In the artisan group most were employed in tailoring and cabinet making and this group increased after 1925, indicating that the Glasgow Jewish students were becoming more representative of the community as a whole (Table 5:7).

It is not possible to compare these figures systematically with the occupational structure of the community as a whole. However, it is likely that the children of the more successful elements in the community would have found it easier to enter university and that they would have been over-represented amongst the Jewish student body. Certainly the professional group were substantially over-represented, for the Jewish clergy in Glasgow were a fairly small group. Nevertheless, the substantial artisan element, forming almost one quarter of the total, illustrated that it was possible for this section of Glasgow Jewry to enter university despite the financial and other obstacles they would have to face.

These findings can be confirmed by identifying the parts of Glasgow where the Jewish medical students lived. The most popular area over the period was the Gorbals, the home of almost one third of all the Jewish medical students. As the Jews began to move out of the Gorbals during the 1920's and 1930's the numbers from the Gorbals began to fall but still represented one sixth of the Jewish students for the 1938 to 1945 period. As Jews moved out of the Gorbals the most popular areas were Battlefield and Shawlands, just a mile or two south. A number also moved to the West End, in the area around Garnethill Synagogue and Glasgow University. However, even this move from the Gorbals to such areas as Pollokshields must be kept in perspective, as most of those in Pollokshields were living in tenemental property on the fringes of that area, rather than in the large villas in the district's centre. The Jewish students were reported as forming a cohesive society with no social class distinctions between the Gorbals students and the others. In fact, many

Table 5:7 Parental Occupations of Glasgow Jewish Medical Students: University of Glasgow

	1895-1945		1925-1945	
	No.	%	No.	%
Professional	18	14.4	11	11.3
Entrepreneurial	29	23.0	21	21.7
Artisan	28	22.2	23	23.7
Clerical, agents	20	15.8	15	15.5
Small business	30	23.8	25	25.8
Unskilled	2	0.8	2	2.0
Total	127	100.0	97	100.0
No entry identified	49	28.0	40	28.8

source: Matriculation Slips, Faculty of Medicine, University of Glasgow
    49 students not identified because father dead, no entry given, or slips not found.

Table 5:8 Home Addresses of Glasgow Jewish Medical Students: University of Glasgow

	1895-1945		1938-1945	
	No.	%	No.	%
Gorbals	40	31.2	6	15.8%
Battlefield	38	30.0	13	34.2%
West End	31	24.4	11	28.8%
Shawlands	9	7.2	5	13.2%
Pollokshields	8	6.4	3	8.0%
Others	1	0.8	-	-
Total	127	100.0	38	100.0

source: Matriculation Slips, Faculty of Medicine, University of Glasgow

of those now resident in areas south of the Gorbals would have been living in the Gorbals only a few years before.[36] Thus, geographically also the Glasgow Jewish medical students were representative of Glasgow Jewry as a whole (Table 5:8).

When the parental occupations are compared with those of the general student body some interesting features can be identified (Table 5:9). The Jewish professional element is much smaller, as one would expect in a community largely of immigrant origins, whose only professional group, that of the ministers of religion, had obtained their qualifications in Eastern Europe. Jews were over-represented in the small business group, and the clerical and agents group and their presence in the entrepreneurial group was similar to that of the general student body. However, it is in the artisan group that the largest difference appears. Students whose fathers were artisans made up 12.4% of medical students in 1929-30 a figure which had increased only

Table 5:9 Parental Occupations of Medical Matriculants, University of Glasgow

	1911-13		1929-30		1926-35	
	No.	%	No.	%	No.	%
Professional	186	34.7	334	34.8	441	32.6
Entrepreneur	133	24.8	197	20.5	217	16.0
Artisan	56	10.4	119	12.4	182	13.4
Clerical, agents	35	6.5	94	9.8	146	10.8
Farmer	11	2.1	16	1.7	22	1.7
Small business	77	14.4	131	13.7	242	18.0
Civil service	12	2.2	32	3.3	53	3.9
Unskilled	6	1.1	23	2.5	45	3.3
Unemployed	-	-	3	0.3	4	0.3
Total	536	100.0	959	100.0	1,352	100.0

source: Adam Collier, 'Social Origins of a Sample of Entrants to Glasgow University', *Sociological Review*, Vol. XXX (1938) pp. 177, 182-3

be claimed that the aim was to improve standards by reducing the numbers of students. The reality was that Jewish students faced new admissions procedures which discriminated against them in subtle ways.

Following Dr. Gavin's remarks in 1929 a national report was conducted by Dr. A. I. Rongy in the *Jewish Tribune* of New York City.[30] He found that while Jews were admitted to medical schools in a percentage fully $3\frac{1}{2}$ times their proportion in the general population, nevertheless the Jewish demand for medical school places was such that only one out of three Jewish applicants was being admitted to medical school. He considered that this was beneficial to the Jewish physician who had, he said, a chiefly Jewish clientèle, and restrictions on Jewish medical students would prevent the development of uneconomic conditions. He recommended that the Jewish community should discourage its young men from studying medicine. However, among Jews already in the professional élite there was a reluctance to intervene on behalf of their co-religionists who were seeking to enter the medical profession. Indeed some of these Jews could display the same hostility to Jewish progress as those applying the quotas.[31]

In December 1930 Dr. Harold Rypins wrote an article on the problem in the 'American Hebrew'.[30] Dr. Rypins pointed out that there were only 6,000 freshman places in medicine while double that number were applying for places. In 1929 the medical schools in New York City had admitted 524 students of whom 226 were Jewish. Jews had made up 76% of the applicants and 43% of the first year admissions. He noted that 17% of all the medical students nationally were Jewish and insisted that the apparent discrimination was explained by the lack of places and geographical factors. However, he did admit that there were a 'very large number of ambitious and capable Jewish students who.......are banned from the study of medicine' and that these students presented a special problem which had to find a solution. Nobody seemed to feel that it was as illogical to oppose the traditional tendency of Jews to enter medicine as to object to Italian dominance of opera, Germans in precision crafts and the Irish in the American police.[32]

The combination of accepting the presence of a certain amount of discrimination and explaining away some of the problem on the grounds that it was in Jewish self-interest, was also taken up by others. Indeed, at a convention of the American Jewish Congress in October 1931 the conclusion was reached that there should be a medical school primarily for Jewish students. Because of the difficulty some Jews faced in entering certain specialities, particulary in surgery, it was also suggested that the Jewish communities should be more active in providing the facilities for Jewish specialists.[33] At the Annual Meeting of the American Jewish Committee held in December 1931 it was felt that because of the fear of medical overcrowding the solution was better vocational guidance for Jewish young men and women about to embark on a professional career.[28] It is interesting that this last view received widespread endorsement in the Jewish press over the next year.

In December 1934 an article appeared in the *Jewish Daily Bulletin* written by Dr. Rongy agreeing that the reduction in the number of Jewish medical students was an economic necessity and pointing to the fact that it was the

Table 6:1 *Numerical Increase in Jewish Physicians Practising in Ten Major American Cities in each quinquenium*

1901-1905	183
1906-1910	256
1911-1915	261
1916-1920	296
1921-1925	513
1926-1930	283
1931-1935	244

(Extrapolated from: Jacob A. Goldberg, 'Jews in the Medical Profession: A National Survey', *Jewish Social Studies* Vol. 1 (1939) p.329.

better qualified Jewish students who were accepted for medical school and that the quotas were not always motivated by anti-Jewish prejudice. Again vocational guidance was seen as one of the answers.[34] During 1934 the AMA made it clear that their response to the American economic crisis which reduced medical incomes was to restrict the supply of doctors rather than amplify medical demand, for example by the encouragement of health insurance. Walter Bierring, incoming president of the A.M.A in 1934, recommended eliminating half the medical schools in the country. Enrolments fell in the six years after 1934 and the Jewish student entry became even more restricted (Tables 6:1 and 6:2).

It was becoming clear that there were discriminatory practices in operation but that their application was being couched in terms which could lead the observer to believe that these restrictions were actually in the best interests of the Jews themselves.[34] The Jewish students themselves were under no illusions about the restrictiveness of the quota and that its application was not solely motivated to provide an increase in the standards of medical students. Some very well qualified students had great difficulty in obtaining admission and there were cases of outstanding students who were being excluded. Julius Axelrod was denied entrance to medical school when he graduated from CCNY in 1933. Instead he turned to biochemistry and went

Table 6:2 *Jewish Students in American Medical Schools 1934-1939*

Year of admission	Schools reporting	Jewish students at schools reporting
1933	75	912
1934	74	836
1935	74	848
1936	72	617
1937	66	587
1938	52	327

source: Jacob A. Goldberg, 'Jews in the Medical Profession: A National Survey', *Jewish Social Studies* Vol. 1 (1939) p.33.

on to win a Nobel Prize in 1970 for his work on the role of certain chemicals in the transmission of nerve impulses.[35] Similarly, George Rosen the doyen of medical historians was denied entry to medical school in the States, not on account of ability, for he was a bright and talented student, but because of the Jewish quota.[36] Rosen and two companions entered the medical faculty of the University of Berlin and in addition to learning German and gaining an interest in medical history, he was uniquely placed to learn of the dangers inherent in the rise of Nazism.

Some of the American Jews who were accepted to the Scottish medical schools knew of highly qualified candidates for medical school who had been denied entry in the States, including those with grades of over 90%.[37] The Jewish students had a particular problem in that few of them could claim 'medical heritage', i.e. a parent who had studied medicine and who might have been able to intercede on the student's behalf. It was also easier for those who had amassed some money and were prepared to supply colleges with endowment funds to get their sons into medical school. For those Jewish students who had studied at college out of New York State there was a possibility that they might be able to proceed to medical school near their college, especially in areas like the midwest.

For those well qualified Jewish college graduates from New York City the difficulties were likely to be greatest. Jews in this group were the likeliest to display greatest hostility to those Jews in positions of leadership within the American medical profession and who did not speak up on their behalf. A particular target was Morris Fishbein, editor of the *Journal of the American Medical Association*, who had acted as the 'token Jew' and had kept silent during the critical period.[37] In a letter to *JAMA* in October 1939 Fishbein wrote that it was 'obvious' that many medical schools were turning down Jewish medical students on racial grounds. At the same time he accepted that Jews now made up over 15% of the medical profession while they only made up about $3\frac{1}{2}$% of the American population.

As an example of the pattern of exclusion practised at medical school, the history of Jewish admissions at Cornell University can be examined. In 1930 the Jewish students made up one quarter of the entering class. In 1940 Dean Ladd stated in writing that there was a Jewish quota of 10-12% and the Jewish acceptances in subsequent years followed so closely to this pattern as to be able to make the inference that the result was clearly related to the effect of introducing the quota. In 1950 less than 5% of suitably qualified Jews were accepted compared with 15.3% of Catholics and 24.6% of Protestants. The figures become all the more remarkable when it is realised that Jewish candidates made up 20 out of the 30 with the highest scholarship grades. Cornell's practice of selecting students from a wide variety of preparatory colleges had the effect of making it difficult to prove discrimination in individual cases.[38]

Even at New York University Medical School and the Long Island Colleges of Medicine, which were more liberal in their attitude to the admission of Jewish students, the percentage of Jewish students dropped from 30-40% in 1920 to less than 20% twenty years later.[39]

While Cornell had a wide catchment area, Columbia was prepared to accept students from a narrower base of colleges which meant that they would have a higher percentage of Jewish students. In fact, Columbia had been the first medical school to introduce selective admission procedures.[40] Jewish students had formed about half of the class in the peak year of 1919. By 1924 the percentage had declined to about 20% although it rose temporarily to around 33% around 1930. After this there was a further downturn during the 1930's which took the figure down to 10-12%. When a local Jewish newspaper commented on the statistics suggesting that there was a quota operating against the Jewish students, the authorities defended themselves by saying that the figures appeared to be based on the results of applications from candidates from CCNY. Dean William Darragh admitted that they were admitting fewer entrants from this college 'not because they are Jews but because they seem to have less desirable qualifications than many of our applicants from other colleges'.[40]

The pattern of discrimination at Yale has been carefully researched.* Prior to 1920 Yale did not have a great reputation as a medical school and it was ironic that its period of greatest success in medicine, co-inciding with the period of the greatest problems for Jewish students in trying to enter medicine, should follow the appointment of a Jewish Dean, Milton Charles Winternitz.[41] Winternitz held the position for fifteen years until 1935 and during that time wrought a most remarkable transformation in the Medical School which opened various new departments and attracted the best medical scientists on to its faculty. The motivation at Yale for maintaining a Jewish quota in the medical school was based on the desire that the white Anglo-Saxon male should continue to hold a monopoly in the medical profession. Winternitz must have been aware of the moves towards quotas in the other major American medical schools at the time of his appointment, and under his leadership Yale would do the same. Winternitz created an admissions committee in 1930 which had detailed instructions: 'Never admit more than five Jews, take only two Italian Catholics and take no blacks at all'.[42] In 1938-9 of 505 applications, 226 or about 45% were from Jewish students. While 26% of the non-Jews were admitted only 3% of the Jews were given places. The quota system continued unabated during the Second World War at Yale, and at other medical schools, so that there was still a 10% Jewish quota in operation in the mid-1940's which operated to the disadvantage of applicants from Brooklyn and the Bronx.[43]

The situation during the early 1930's was difficult enough but it became even harder for Jewish medical students after 1937 with a further drop in Jewish enrolments in medical school by 40%. With war limiting the ability of American Jews to come to Scotland and other overseas medical schools, the position was actually becoming more acute. The discrimination was becoming so entrenched that it was hardly being questioned any more.[44] The predominately Jewish graduates of CCNY found great difficulty in finding

---

*Dan Oren, *Joining the Club* (1985).

places in the major medical colleges and the percentage of CCNY graduates entering medical school fell from 58% in 1925 and 34% in 1932 to only about 15% between 1939 and 1943. While three quarters of non-Jewish applicants were being accepted, amongst Jews the proportion was one in thirteen.

Statistics could therefore be employed both by the college authorities as well as by the Jews to prove their own particular viewpoint. However, such figures might indicate a general problem in obtaining places but it did not indicate where and how the problems might arise.[40] This was especially the case in medical schools, the authorities were not as forthcoming as the Deans of Cornell and Columbia. Lawrence Bloomgarden's *Preliminary Analysis of Discrimination Against Jewish Applicants for Admission to Medical Schools in New York State* furnished detailed evidence showing the continuation of Jewish quotas beyond 1940, when they were acknowledged, and even into the postwar period.

As the full implications of the effects of the Holocaust in Europe was revealed after the Second World War, overt anti-semitism was on the decline. Restrictive admissions began to yield slowly to public criticism after the Second World War[45] particularly under pressure from returning Jewish veterans. Nevertheless, there remained evidence of continuing discrimination through the 1950's and it was not until the 1960's that the quota system had been finally abandoned. By 1956 there was reported to be a three to four-fold increase in Jewish enrolment at the medical colleges.

From these illustrations it is possible to discern some anti-Jewish discrimination in the application of entrance procedures at some of the American medical schools. While Jewish students were not alone in facing discrimination they showed the greatest ingenuity in trying to find alternative ways to achieve their ambitions. Many undoubtedly gave up their dreams of entering the medical profession choosing instead other areas of medical science. A number became dentists and it was said in Stamford, Connecticut that D.D.S. stood for 'disappointed doctor or surgeon'.[46] A few Italians found their way back to Italy to study medicine but for the rejected, and dejected Jew, the way abroad to Switzerland, Scotland or Germany proved to be the simplest solution and became increasingly popular during the 1930's.[47] Reports from returning Jewish students and other sources indicated that about 90% of American students abroad were Jewish,[48] and the figure was even higher if the Italian medical schools are excluded.

For many American Jews the reason for coming to Scotland was simple. They had applied to many, sometimes to dozens, of medical schools in America and they could not find a place. Brighter students should, theoretically, have had less difficulty in finding a place in America but even some of the best Jewish students could not always manage to gain acceptance. For the more average Jewish student a place in one of the American medical schools based on equality of opportunity was simply not available. The only possibility, if medicine was to remain the career choice, was to seek to study elsewhere.

For other students the flexibility of entrance qualifications in Scotland enabled intending medical students to take a wider range of subjects at college. Some only decided they wanted to do medicine after study at college, and without a background in the sciences they found that Scotland indeed offered the solution to their problems. There were advantages to study in Scotland over continental destinations. Firstly there were the traditional links with Scotland which had existed since colonial times, with Scottish medicine being held in high respect. In addition, the English language was a powerful factor making the choice of Scotland more attractive. Naturally as the wave of anti-semitism in Europe increased during the 1930's Germany, Italy and Austria became less popular (Tables 6:3-6:5).

American interest in medical study in Britain can be identified from about 1926. This trend came to the attention of the General Medical Council during 1930 when it was stated that over 250 prospective American students had been turned away from the Universities of Birmingham and Manchester with no reason given.[49] A memorandum was prepared by the Registrar of the Council on the question of American medical students. The Americans had registered their concern about the matter because they felt that if students who had been deemed unsuitable in the States could obtain qualifications abroad then difficulties over medical standards would ensue. It was acknowledged that those seeking places in Britain had varying levels of qualifications and it was agreed that it was important to ensure that any Americans admitted to British medical schools should have attained an adequate standard in their pre-clinical studies in college.

After some correspondence between the General Medical Council and the National Board of Medical Examiners in the States, it was agreed that students intending to enter medical school in Britain should show evidence of their eligibility by producing a satisfactory collegiate record. It had been acknowledged by Dean Rappleye, who had been present at meetings of the General Medical Council in May 1930, that in fact the most common reason for students not being accepted into American medical schools was that the schools were being designated as 'class full'. This was said to be the least objectionable designation by which students can be rejected for personal or racial grounds.[49]

Table 6:3   Citizens of the U.S.A. Enrolled in Faculties of Medicine Abroad

	30-31	32-33	34-35	36-37	38-39
Austria	114	271	235	185	-
England	52	57	78	47	36
France	25	78	89	40	18
Germany	72	439	246	245	45
Ireland	14	20	6	7	9
Italy	78	282	286	265	54
Scotland	256	416	476	386	401
Switzerland	65	405	396	316	56
Others	34	84	125	140	61
Total	710	2052	1937	1631	680

from JAMA Vol. 113 (1939) p.772

Table 6:4 Medical Licensure Statistics for 1933-1937

	No. Examined	% Failed
Universitat Wien	200	27.5
Universite de Paris	75	33.3
Freidrich-Wilhems Universitat (Berlin)	180	31.7
Ludwig-Maximillians Universitat (Munchen)	62	27.4
Regia Universita di Napoli	134	61.9
Regia Universeita di Roma	188	49.5
Universitat Bern	127	35.4
Universitat Basel	63	27.0
Universitat Zurich	66	27.3
Universite de Geneve	66	27.3
Scottish Universities	208	10.0
Scottish Triple Qualification	135	20.0
ITALY	451	54.4
SWITZERLAND	368	30.3
AUSTRIA	228	29.4
ENGLAND	93	16.1
SCOTLAND	343	14.1

source: *JAMA* Vol. 112 (1939) p.1721

The General Medical Council realised that it was treading on dangerous ground as the Medical Act did not cover admission to medical school in the pre-clinical stage and the Council did not wish to interfere with the prerogatives of the British medical schools. Concern was also expressed that in view of the reciprocal arrangements in existence that British Medical Schools should not permit Americans to obtain their qualifications in a shorter time than would have been possible in the States.

The Scottish Branch of the General Medical Council also had several meetings during 1930 to discuss admission procedures for the American appli-

Table 6:5 American Medical Students in Scotland: 1930-1939

	American Medical Students in Scotland	Total Americans Studying Medicine Abroad	% in Scotland
1930-1931	256	710	36.1
1931-1932	286	1206	23.7
1932-1933	416	2052	20.2
1933-1934	444	1903	23.3
1934-1935	476	1937	24.6
1935-1936	369	1637	22.5
1936-1937	386	1631	23.7
1937-1938	525	1298	40.5
1938-1939	401	680	59.0

from *JAMA* Vol. 113 (1939) p.772

cants. At one of these meetings Dr. J. S. Rodman, Secretary of the National Board of Medical Examiners of the U.S.A., was present by invitation. It was recommended that all applications from America for admission to Medical Schools in Scotland should be forwarded to the Registrar of the Scottish Branch Council for verification of authenticity. It was noted at the November meeting of the Scottish Branch in 1930 that some 20 Americans had applied under the new arrangements and had been accepted to study.[49]

These arrangements proved satisfactory and in the Presidential Address to the General Medical Council reported in the 1932 minutes, it was stated that the previous difficulties had almost completely disappeared and that the Council was particularly indebted to Dr. Zapffe, of the Association of American Medical Colleges, for his 'untiring help in regard to verifications and evaluation of certificates'.[50] The President was also pleased to note the cordial references in the Assocation's own journal in the States to the part played by the General Medical Council in dealing with these matters.

The large majority of Americans studying in Britain came to Scotland with the Scottish preponderance increasing through the 1930's. The links between the Scottish medical schools and North America are of longstanding and predate the founding of the American medical schools. Edinburgh especially had a close link with the new medical schools founded in North America and many of the first teachers there were Edinburgh graduates. Indeed the first Jews to graduate in medicine in both Edinburgh and Glasgow were Americans. As time went on and the American system of medical education became more established, it was still not uncommon for the sons of Scottish graduates to return to Edinburgh and Glasgow to pursue their medical studies. Thus there was still a custom of American medical students at Edinburgh University continuing into the twentieth century. However this small and traditional link was gradually overwhelmed by the large numbers of American Jews seeking places to study in Scotland when they discovered that it was not possible to study in their native land.

The pattern of American students studying in Scotland appears to bear this out. The geographical origins of the Jewish students from America shows the preponderance of students from the North Eastern States, in particular from New York and New Jersey. For non-Jewish American medical students in Scotland there is a different geographical pattern with fewer students from New York and a wide distribution from all over America (Table 6:6).

Jewish students were irritated by the attempts of the American medical authorities to denigrate their standards and to try and deny them the opportunity of studying abroad, while removing their chances of studying at home.

The prevailing American attitude was that overseas students were 'second rate'. Thus the exclusion of many talented students was justified on the basis of improving standards. However, an examination of the educational records of the Americans in Scotland does not confirm this suggestion. In St. Andrews the American students obtained the share of class medals and first class certificates that would be expected from the relative numbers. In the University of Glasgow some exceptional candidates were enrolled. In 1934[51] the Brunton Prize for the most distinguished graduate went to Robert Elitzik of

Table 6:6 *Geographical Distribution of American Medical Students and Graduates in Scotland 1925-1940*

	All American Jewish Graduates		American Jewish Students at Anderson College		All American non-Jewish Graduates	
New York	152	89%	771	90%	10	36%
New Jersey	12	7%	39	5%	6	21%
Pennsylvania	3	2%	22	3%	1	4%
others	4	2%	15	2%	11	39%
Total	171	100%	847	100%	28	100%

New York and the West of Scotland Prize went to Emmanuel Rappaport, also of New York.[52] These two graduated with honours and four other Americans graduated with commendation, a high percentage of the 13 Americans. These findings of exceptional intellectual ability were confirmed by contemporary students in all the university centres and by the Medical School of the Royal Colleges in Edinburgh. In 1931 the Colleges' Medical School had received a letter from Dr. Zappfe, Secretary of the Association of American Medical Colleges, seeking information on American students in Scotland and expressing the opinion that the American applicants to British medical schools were of the very lowest educational standard and not likely to be admitted into any, even the least, of the American Schools. The Dean was instructed to reply giving the desired information and indicating that in the opinion of the lecturers the quality of the American students presenting themselves was not in accordance with Dr. Zappfe's opinion. On the contrary the feeling was that the American students, in quite a number of occasions, headed the class examination lists.[53]

During the 1930's there were changes in the pattern of American student attendance at the various Scottish medical schools. The initial preference for the universities gradually gave way, based on more favourable admissions policies, to an overwhelming concentration in the extra-mural medical schools (Table 6:7).

It will be seen that this shift from the universities to the extra-mural medical schools came about for a number of reasons. There was first of all the sheer size of the number of applications relative to the number of places likely to be left unfilled by local candidates. The universities maintained an entry of American students through the early 1930's and it was only the number of American applications which led to the introduction of a more restrictive policy. In Edinburgh too it was the sheer weight of numbers which led to the introduction of a consistent policy for the admission of overseas students. Nevertheless, no discrimination against Jews can be identified as all suitably qualified Scottish Jews, who wished to do so, were able to study medicine.

The flexibility of the extra-mural colleges and their ability to expand rapidly to meet the needs of the increasing numbers of newcomers enabled them to

Table 6:7 Place of Enrolment of 1st Year American Jewish Medical Students in Scotland: 1925-1938

	Univ. of Glasgow	Univ. of Edinburgh	Univ. of Aberdeen	Univ. of St. Andrews	Extra-mural Medical Colleges*
1925		2			
1926		13		3	
1927		13		6	1
1928	2	2	1	31	18
1929	13	3	9	22	10
1930	4	5	1	12	31
1931	10	5		6	39
1932	1	8	1	3	41
1933		3		1	55
1934					56
1935					80
1936					76
1937					64
1938					66

Source: Matriculation Albums of the Scottish Medical Schools
*From 1936 Anderson's College only.

compete successfully in the market for American students. Considered in strict financial terms it was the skillful entrepreneurial policy of the extra-mural schools which paved the way for their remarkable levels of admission during the 1930's but it may have been this very success which was to lead to their abolition after the Second World War.

At the University of Glasgow there were 23 American applicants for the 1928-1929 session. In January 1929 it was decided to fix the capacity of the medical school at 200 per annum and as numbers fell below this level over the next three or four sessions it was possible to admit a number of Americans, between 7 and 15, each year. By 1932 the number of American applications was rising steadily and there was a clear need for a more critical selection policy. The Clerk to the Faculty, who was processing an increasing number of applications, was instructed in November 1932 that with a limited number of places and increasing demand from home students there was no likelihood of overseas students being accepted. Senate records show that 66 Americans applied in 1932 and that 250 foreign applications were received in 1935 without specifying country of origin.[54]

The admissions policy in Edinburgh University differed only slightly. The topic of American admissions was first discussed in 1928 when the Medical Faculty set up a committee to discuss the question. This committee functioned as a clearing house for the processing of applications and did not adjudicate on the question of whether foreign students should be admitted. The committee finally made a report in 1934 and there was agreement on limiting annual admissions to 220. Preference for overseas admissions was to be given to students from the Colonies, especially from areas like the British West

Indies, which did not have a medical school of their own. There was to be a limit of 10% on students from Commonwealth countries like Australia, New Zealand, South Africa and India. Students would be admitted from China if 'well qualified' and from Egypt and the United States if 'exceptionally well qualified'. Thus a few Americans continued to be admitted.

In St. Andrews University a considerable number of Americans studied medicine from 1927. The peak year for American graduates was 1933 when 31 out of the 46 graduands were American, and all but two of them were from New York or New Jersey. In the 10 years preceding the first graduation of Americans, St. Andrews medical classes had been very small, with on average less than 30 doctors graduating each year. However, even after the number of Americans in St. Andrews declined the University was able to maintain its increased number of medical students. This remarkably large group of American students, who studied in St. Andrews and took their clinical course in Dundee, formed almost one third of all the medical students between 1932 and 1937. It is thought that Sir James Irvine, who was a frequent visitor to the States, encouraged the Americans to come when he learned of the difficulties prospective Jewish medical students were facing.[51] New Yorkers were also attracted by a Scottish science lecturer at New York University.[55] Frank Charteris, then Dean of the Medical Faculty, was also supportive of the Americans and he nurtured their attachment to the University.[55] The American graduates showed their appreciation by forming the St. Andrews American Medical Alumni Association which has raised thousands of dollars for St. Andrews University and endowed scholarships and provided other academic support.

The primary consideration in Aberdeen was the provision of places for local students although a group of eleven Americans was admitted in 1928. The rising level of local applicants meant that not all qualified applicants from the Aberdeen area could be admitted. In 1930 alone Aberdeen University received no less than 203 medical applications from America, with virtually all the candidates graduates of the College of the City of New York and New York University.

Thus the Scottish Universities coped with the influx of Americans to the best of their abilities and in far greater numbers and for a far longer period than the English universities were able to do. Their response included the high levels of Americans who studied at St. Andrews and Dundee, and in Glasgow and Edinburgh the reduction in numbers of Americans followed the level of American applications continuing at a level far beyond their ability to admit. The Edinburgh response had been to institute a carefully balanced international student policy while Glasgow, with its larger local population base, gave preference to local candidates. However, the American students did not suffer from this re-organising of priorities as the extra-mural medical colleges both in Glasgow and in Edinburgh were well able to fill the gap.

Of the three Scottish extra-mural schools the smallest was St. Mungo's College, based on the Glasgow Royal Infirmary.[56] The Medical Faculty there were concerned with their low level of enrolments, with less than 100 students in 1927-8. They considered amalgamation with Anderson's College,

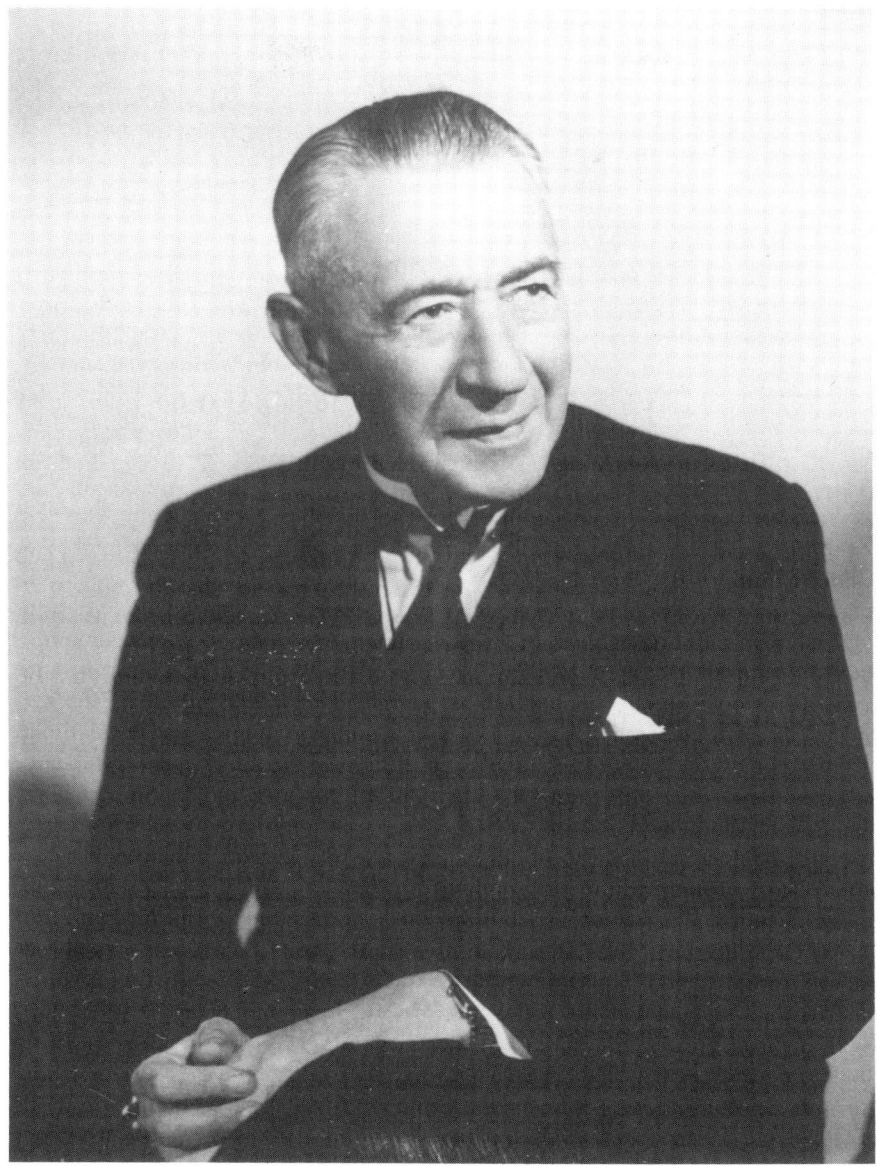

24 Sir James Irvine, Principal of St Andrews University.

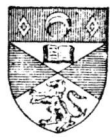

ST. ANDREWS UNIVERSITY MEDICAL SCHOOL.

MAY, 1930.

FROM THE DEAN,

MEDICAL FACULTY. To Herbert Goldberg

Dear Sir

I am prepared to admit you into the First year group of the medical school in Dundee for the session commencing October 2nd 1930. Please let me know as soon as possible whether you are able to accept this offer.

Yours faithfully,

J. V. Charters
Dean

25 Certificate of acceptance for entry to the Medical School in Dundee, October 1930.

the other Glasgow extra-mural school, but Anderson's College were not in favour of such a move. With the arrival of the Americans the student roll began to increase rapidly. In 1936-7 St. Mungo's agreed to admit about 100 Americans for the winter and summer sessions and to charge them a deposit of £5.

Anderson's College, which was based on Glasgow's Western Infirmary, was a larger institution than St. Mungo's. Some university students were attracted to classes where the teaching was of an exceptionally high standard, such as in anatomy and physiology. Despite the huge influx of Americans to Anderson's College, the numbers reaching over 250 in 1938, there are no records in the College Minutes concerning the admission of the Americans. The University of Glasgow was alarmed at the strain the number of foreign students was placing on teaching facilities in the city and it suggested in 1937 that the extra-mural colleges adopt the same admission policy as the university (Table 6:8).

These figures are complicated because some students commenced studies in Second Year and there was some interchange with St. Mungo's College. Nevertheless it confirms the steady progression of American students through their undergraduate studies and shows that only a small number of students dropped out.

Anderson's College and St. Mungo's College both decided not to admit any Americans for the session commencing in October 1939 but the outbreak of war meant that no new students were able to arrive anyway. There was continuing resentment amongst the honorary clinical staff at the University about the success of the extra-mural colleges in recruiting so many foreign students with the accompanying prosperity this implied. Extra-mural college

Table 6:8   American Jewish Medical Students at Anderson's College, Glasgow

YEAR	1st	2nd	3rd	4th	5th	Total
1925	—	—	—	—	—	—
1926	—	—	—	—	—	—
1927	1	—	—	—	—	1
1928	—	—	—	—	—	—
1929	1	2	—	—	—	3
1930	10	14	—	—	—	24
1931	20	15	4	—	1	40
1932	18	27	7	11	3	66
1933	20	22	12	11	6	71
1934	46	17	6	11	9	89
1935	50	43	12	12	6	123
1936	66	47	34	12	9	168
1937	41	79	33	34	9	196
1938	28	73	64	56	32	253
1939	—	3	9	22	19	53
1940	—	—	5	10	11	26

source: Matriculation album, Anderson's College

lecturers received class fees from their students and handed a proportion over to the college authorities.

The Medical School of the Royal Colleges of Edinburgh also based its considerable student enrolment on recruitment of foreign students. In 1932 the 36 Americans were only 4 less than the British students, while there were also some Egyptian, Chinese, South African and Indian students. In 1930 the Medical School developed a system for the processing of American applications, ensuring that the Americans had the correct entry qualifications. While they would supply information on American students' admissions to the American medical authorities, they reserved for themselves the full responsibility for admissions. The Medical School continued to admit substantial numbers of Americans through the 1930's and did not suffer any limitation in numbers following discussions with the University about the maximum medical teaching capacity in the city. Over the years the extramural medical school in Edinburgh became a less popular choice than the colleges in Glasgow. It may have been due to Glasgow's greater size and larger Jewish community and as the Glasgow numbers increased the students attracted there would have encouraged their friends and associates from America to follow them to Glasgow. However, the outbreak of war in 1939 ended the influx of Americans to Edinburgh (Table 6:9).

In 1939 Dean Willard Rappleye, Director of Studies of the Commission on Medical Education of the American Medical Colleges toured Europe to inspect medical institutions at which Americans were studying medicine. There was some resentment in Edinburgh that Scottish medical institutions were being manipulated as an agency of American medical politics. Dr. John Orr, Dean of the School of Medicine of the Royal Colleges in Edinburgh, in a letter to the American Medical Club in Glasgow, made it clear that he regarded the inspection of his School, which had lasted merely one hour, as representing something 'very sinister' and he considered that racial discrimination entered largely into the question.[57] He could hardly believe otherwise, with an American student body both large and almost exclusively Jewish.[58]

The English medical schools appear to have taken firmer action to enforce the suggestions of the General Medical Council that caution be exercised in

Table 6:9   Place of Study of Americans Taking Triple Qualification

	Glasgow	Edinburgh	Total
1933	1	17	18
1934	2	8	10
1935	12	17	29
1936	16	23	39
1937	15	26	41
1938	18	33	51
1939	31	23	54
1940	53	28	81
Total	148	175	323

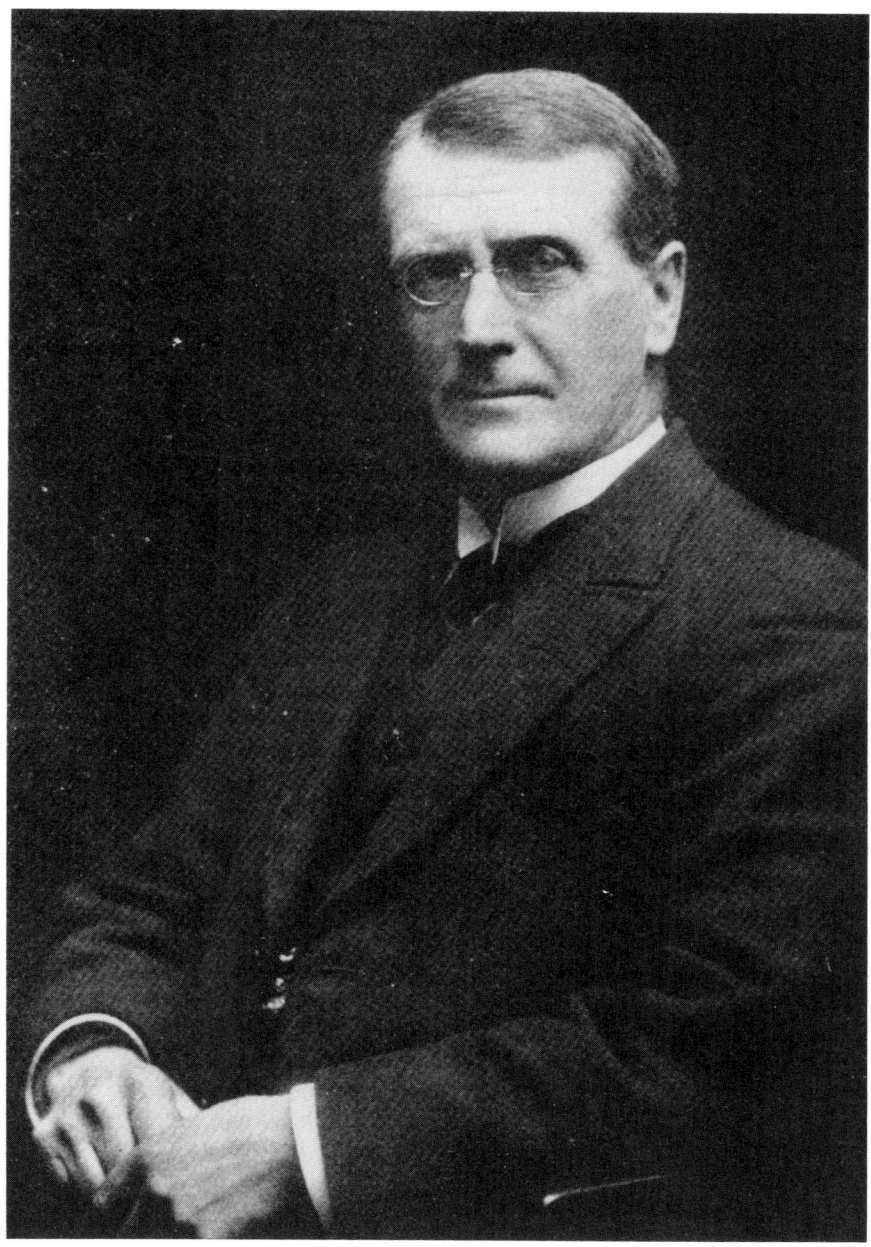

26 John Orr, Dean of the Medical School of the Royal Colleges, Edinburgh.

the admission of Americans. Following correspondence with the General Medical Council in 1930, Leeds University decided not to admit American medical students. Liverpool University admitted only one American undergraduate to their Medical Faculty during the 1930's. In London a few Americans were admitted to St. Bartholomew's, King's College and Charing Cross and Westminster. This last school was admitting many students from countries such as India, Egypt and South Africa. It may have seemed more prudent to continue admitting students from these traditional overseas countries rather than get involved in medico-political arguments over the admission of Americans.

By comparison, the Scottish medical schools, particularly the extra-mural colleges and to a lesser extent the universities, were showing a combination of practical sympathy and traditional entrepreneurial skill. The extra-mural schools benefitted from the influx of Americans and increased their rolls quite substantially. This was sufficient to put Scotland on the map as the major overseas centre for the training of American born physicians during the 1930's.

Some American medical students who had not completed their courses by 1939 were dismayed by the news that the New York and New Jersey Boards of Examiners planned to stop recognition of the Scottish Triple Qualification, which was the final examination of the extra-mural colleges. However, it was subsequently made clear that the ruling was not retrospective and would not apply to students who had already started their courses in Scotland.[59]

Students who were in America for the summer vacation in 1939 were faced with the prospect of being refused permission to return to Scotland to complete their studies as the U.S. State Department had discontinued the issuing of visas to combat areas.[60] Following popular pressure from the specially formed American Medical Clubs of Scotland and supported by the Mayor of New York and other personalities, it was agreed late in 1939 that students in the last two years of their studies should be allowed to return to Scotland. Fifty students returned to Scotland but there were more than 300, who were at earlier stages of their course, who were unable to do so. A number of them did manage to find places in America or in neutral Switzerland. By the 1950's there were only a handful of American medical students in Scotland. For those Americans who completed their studies in Scotland during the war it was not easy to return to the States and many took jobs in Britain until the end of the war.

The numbers of Americans taking the Triple Qualification fell from 80 in 1940 to 27 in 1942 and then averaged about 10 over the next five years. The Americans studying in Scotland had a good record in passing State Board examinations on return home. The best results were obtained by Glasgow University's American graduates who achieved 100% success in New York State Board examinations (Tables 6:10-6:11).

The Medical School of the Royal Colleges of Edinburgh also referred to the 'racial question as affecting the Jewish race' in their comments on the Goodenough Commission on Medical Education which recommended the closure of the extra-mural schools after the war.[61] They rebutted the claims

Table 6:10   Medical Licensure Statistics for 1938

	1933-1937		1938	
	No. exam.	% failed	No. exam.	% failed
England				
LMSSA	5	60.0	0	0
LRCP, MRCS	59	10.2	0	0
Univ.of Birmingham	3	0.0	0	0
Univ.of Bristol	1	0.0	1	0
Univ.of Cambridge	1	0.0	0	0
Univ.of Durham, Newcastle	8	25.0	0	0
Univ.of Liverpool	1	0.0	0	0
Univ.of London	8	37.5	0	0
Univ.of Oxford	1	0.0	0	0
Univ.of Sheffield	6	16.7	3	0
Ireland				
LRCPI, LRCSI	3	0.0	1	100
National Univ.of Ireland	6	16.7	2	50
Univ. of Dublin	11	27.3	2	50
Scotland				
LRCP&S(Ed.), LRFPS(Glas)	135	20.0	61	19.7
Univ. of Aberdeen	14	14.3	0	0
Univ. of Edinburgh	66	10.6	4	0
Univ. of Glasgow	32	0.0	7	0
Univ. of St. Andrews	96	12.5	4	0
Total				
England	93	16.1	4	0
Ireland	20	20.0	5	60.0
Scotland	343	14.0	76	14.5
Total	456		85	

source: JAMA 112 (1939) p.1721

made about the American students, namely that they had been excluded from places in the United States in an attempt to improve standards. Dean Orr was aware of developments in America after his visits to universities there in 1930 and 1931. He rejected the view that the Colleges were providing a 'Scottish back-door to the medical profession in the United States'. The records of the graduates of the extra-mural schools in the New York State Board Examinations showed the level of their ability and their training.

Table 6:11   NEW YORK STATE BOARD 1937-8

Students from	examined	passed	%
New York State	488	462	94.5
Scotland	76	63	82.9
Canada	62	51	82.3
U.S.A. (except N.Y.)	285	214	75.1

source: JAMA 112 (1939) p.1721.

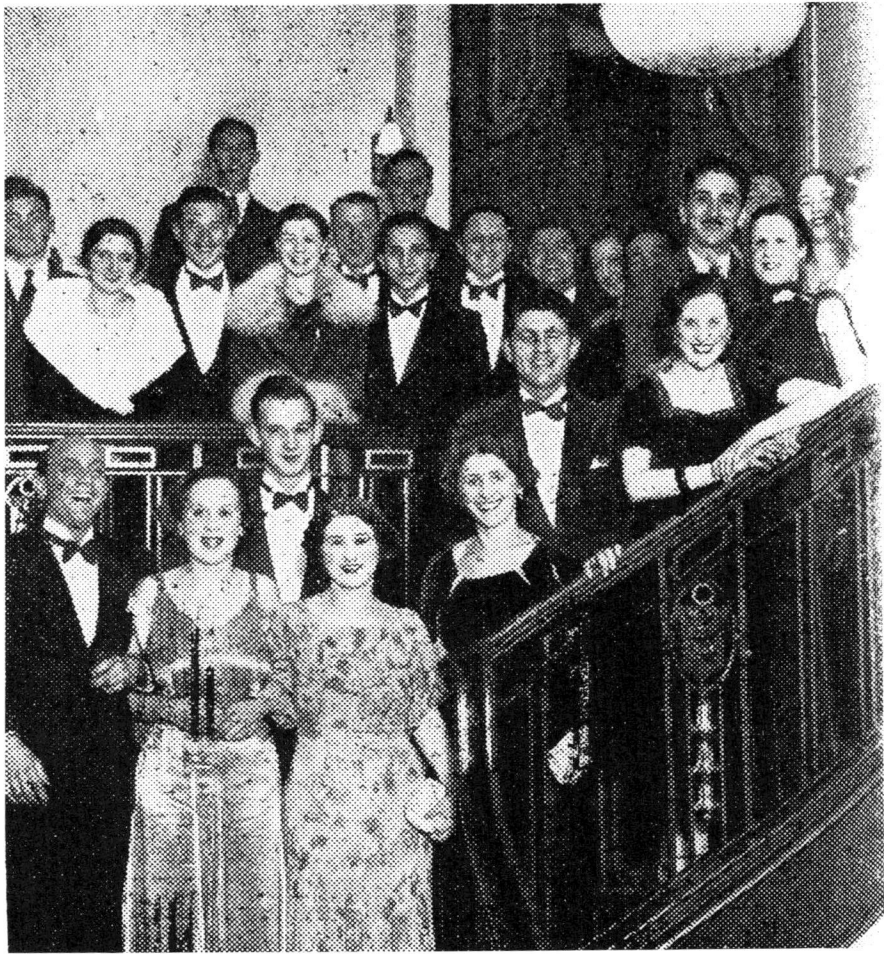

27 Group at the dance held by American medical students at the Marlborough House, Glasgow, November 1935.

The undergraduate experiences and subsequent graduate careers of the Scottish trained American Jewish doctors can be studied employing the analysis of the replies to the questionnaires sent to 120 Scottish graduates of the 1930-1945 period on the 1982 American Medical Directory. The 41 replies, a response rate of 34%, were supplemented by 18 personal interviews conducted on a visit to the United States in March and April 1986.

This showed that for those turned down by medical schools in New York State the costs of study at private schools out of New York State were often prohibitive. By contrast the costs of study in Scotland were quite acceptable, even when all the costs were taken into account. The round trip from the States cost about $100 and some students managed to return to America each summer to keep in contact with their families, but also to have the prospect of earning some money during the long vacation which would help to cover the expenses they would incur during their next year. The cost of digs varied depending on the quality of accommodation and facilities on offer, but 30/- ($7.50) per week is the average figure. Some however paid about 25/- while the more expensive digs cost up to £2 per week. For this sum the student would receive a Scottish breakfast and evening meal and pre-bedtime cup of cocoa in addition to the basic accommodation.

The average monthly expenses totalled about £15 ($75) and this figure was a fairly tight one, not permitting much in the way of luxury. There were some students who had a larger budget but the majority were conscious of the financial sacrifice being made by their families to enable them to study medicine abroad and they were careful with their funds. Herbert Goldberg recalled that his father died during his studies and his mother started a candy business with a friend which helped to raise the $1300 needed to finance each year of studies. There were other methods of saving funds and some students managed to find clinical clerkships which provided free board and lodgings in return for some modest clinical work usually in psychiatric hospitals. The accommodation in St. Andrews was often superior to that found in Glasgow or Edinburgh as it was often used for the tourist trade while the Americans were back home in the summer.

The Americans were recalled as 'wealthy' by fellow-students in Scotland but the situation was not as simple as that. While they were not as dependent on parental funds or Carnegie grants as their Scottish peers, they did have a budget to work to but their American budget may have stretched further than the average Scottish student could afford. Some of the students were married when they came over and they therefore had to finance family accommodation. Failing an examination was unthinkable and the Americans were well motivated to study.

Only a few of the Americans took Jewish digs. Some of the first students who came over made a greater attempt to make contact with the Jewish community as their numbers were smaller and they did not yet have a self-contained society of their own. Belle Shedrowitz recalls being 'ordered' to stay with a Jewish family in Dundee and a number of Americans both in Glasgow and Edinburgh stayed with Jewish families, often with Jewish class-mates beginning friendships that were to endure for many decades. Not all the Jewish digs worked out well. Some students complained about the price, which was perhaps pitched higher to cover the extra costs of kosher food, and some Jewish landladies were upset by the disregard for Orthodox Jewish practices displayed by the Americans. They objected to the American students smoking on the Sabbath and their lack of attendance in the synagogue and even their craving for 'bacon and eggs'.[62]

When the American students first arrived there was an enthusiastic welcome in the Jewish communities in both Edinburgh and Glasgow and local families, especially those with eligible daughters, offered mealtime hospitality.

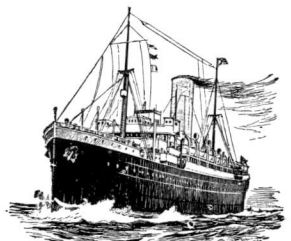

28 Regular trans-Atlantic travel attracted this advertisement to Surgeon's Hall Journal, January–March 1938.

Jesse Holland remembered one Yom Kippur being invited to several different Jewish families in Edinburgh to break the fast. Not wishing to offend anyone by choosing a meal with another family, he went instead to a Chinese restaurant! However, few of the American Jews were religiously observant. In Glasgow they enjoyed the community centre and sporting facilities offered by the Jewish Institute over the other Jewish groups in the city. In 1935 the American Club in Glasgow upset the local Jewish community by holding a dance on Friday evening, on the commencement of the Jewish Sabbath.[62] They protested that they were an American Club and that in fact most of those present were members of the Glasgow Jewish community rather than Americans. The Editor of the *Jewish Echo* pointed out that the vast majority of the members of the American Medical Club, and including all its office-bearers, were Jewish and to say that the Club was not Jewish was 'pure American humbug'.

As the numbers of Americans rose steeply in the late 1930's the Americans became more of a self-enclosed group and there was less contact with local society, both Jewish and non-Jewish. Some today feel that they could have got more out of their time in Scotland by mixing less with their fellow Americans but it is clear that most of those in Scotland in the late 1930's recall little contact with the Jewish community other than visiting the food shops to buy Jewish delicacies or to get a Jewish meal at Geneen's Hotel. To counteract this potential isolation the Glasgow Bnai Brith were holding regular receptions for the Americans by 1938 and made sure that hospitality was being extended to Jewish festivals, especially to Passover.[63] There were inter-meetings between the American Clubs in Glasgow and Edinburgh and the local Jewish Students' Societies and the Americans were active in local sporting activities.

The American medical students introduced baseball into Britain and established a baseball league during the 1930's. Harold Klein also recalled playing rugby football to American football rules and this was greatly enjoyed. In Dundee, where the number of Americans was smaller, there was no formal American Club but they managed to meet regularly and informally, usually at lunchtimes and at the weekends. Herbert Goldberg remembered some students trying to act 'British' and trying to avoid the other Americans.

With many of the Americans on a tight financial budget difficulties were bound to arise. Two brothers who studied in Edinburgh and were notorious for their lack of money, managed to solve their problems when one brother was befriended by the aunt of a former girl-friend who helped to support him through the remainder of his studies. The Glasgow Jewish Board of Guardians were reluctant to get involved in giving aid to the Americans though one or two did try to obtain funds from them. The Board felt that those who could travel half way round the world to study should not be a charge on the meagre resources available for the Jewish poor in the hungry years of the 1930's.

In Edinburgh, the American students were aware of Rabbi Salis Daiches even if they were not regular worshippers in the Synagogue in Salisbury Road. Rabbi Daiches took a keen interest in the problems facing Jewish students seeking a medical education and brought up the matter for discussion with the authorities at the Medical School of the Royal College of Surgeons.[64] He was on friendly terms with Dean John Orr and while his name does not appear in the official minutes his influence certainly cannot be discounted.

Nathaniel Solomon remembered the visit of the Vilna Troupe, the great performers of the Yiddish theatre, to Edinburgh in 1934 when they performed 'Dos Pintele Yid' to a very sparse audience. The actors were displeased with the turn-out and took out their resentment on those present. The students said that they usually tried to date Jewish girls and there are quite a number of marriages which took place between the American students and Jewish girls in Dundee, Edinburgh and Glasgow. However, it took some time for the community to adjust to the flood of Jewish students into their midst. Both Glasgow and Edinburgh had upwards of 250 Americans each by 1938, a very substantial number especially for the Edinburgh Jewish community which numbered about 400 families. The Americans were in town for about eight months of the year and were in Scotland only for a few years.

In Glasgow most of the Americans found digs in the area around the university where the more prosperous Garnethill Hebrew Congregation members lived. Some took lodgings with Jewish families in the poorer Jewish area of the Gorbals. Paul Steinlauf recalled working for the Jewish Board of Guardians helping with the distribution of Passover food to needy families and being surprised at the extent of Jewish poverty in Glasgow, even in the supposedly more prosperous West End. The Americans also attracted many

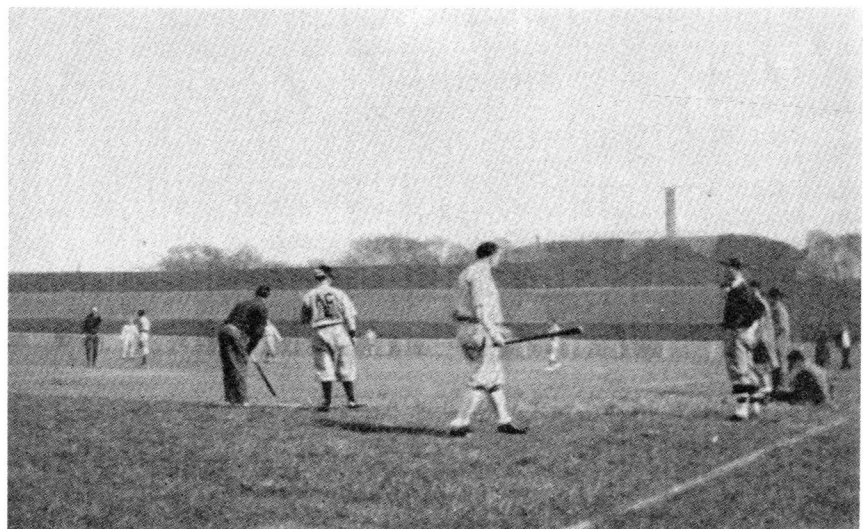

29 American medical students introduced baseball to Scotland. This game was played at Springfield Park, Glasgow 1937.

Edinburgh					Glasgow				
Name	At Bat	Hits	Runs	Errors	Name	At Bat	Hits	Runs	Errors
A. Rosenblatt cf	3	0	0	0	H. Tulipan ss	3	0	1	0
W. Lubansky c	3	1	2	0	J. Greenfield lf	3	0	1	0
H. Michaelson 2nd	3	1	2	0	S. Silverman cf	3	1	3	0
J. Washington 3rd	3	0	1	0	S. Amsterdam 2nd	3	3	2	0
L. Feit lf	3	2	1	0	S. Olansky c	3	3	0	0
A. Taterka 1st	3	0	0	0	D. Skudowitz 3rd	3	1	0	0
G. Blueglass rf	3	0	0	0	P. Margolis rf	2	0	0	0
M. Dillon ss	3	1	0	0	M. Tischler 1st	2	0	1	0
J. Pomerantz p	2	0	0	0	H. Cohen p	2	0	1	0
Substitutions:					*Substitutions:*				
F. Mahoney lf	1	0	0	0	W. Goldstein p	1	0	0	0
H. Berger cf	1	0	0	0	R. Itskowitz 1st	1	0	0	0
C. Abraham 2nd	0	0	0	0	A. Goldstein rf	1	0	0	0
R. Millon lf	0	0	0	0					
Total	28	5	6	0	Total	27	8	9	0

Score by innings:	1	2	3	4	5	Total
Edinburgh	3	0	1	2	0	= 6
Glasgow	2	6	1	0	X	= 9

Game called at end of fifth innings because of time agreement

Substitutions:
Edinburgh: 3rd: Pomerantz out. Dillon to pitch. Blueglass to short. Mahoney to right field.
4th: Taterka, Lubansky and Blueglass out. Shifted Michaelson to 1st, Feit to catcher, Rosenblatt to short. Abraham sent in to 2nd, Millon to left field, and Berger to centre field.
Glasgow: 3rd: Cohen out, Goldstein in the box.
4th: Itskowitz for Tischler at 1st. A. Goldstein to right field for Margolis.
5th: Shifted Amsterdam to pitcher and Goldstein to second.

30 Score-card of the Glasgow–Edinburgh baseball game played by American medical students, 1937.

non-Jewish friends. Some found they were able to mix easily and openly in non-Jewish society including areas where Jewish Scots would have found it difficult to penetrate. American students frequented the Dunedin Palais in Edinburgh and many friendships began there. There were some non-Jewish girls who converted to Judaism and led typically Jewish lives on going with their husbands to the States. A number of other Americans married out of their faith and took their Scottish brides back to America often to a hostile reception from their families in New York.

While Harold Klein, like most others, described his digs in Edinburgh as having been comfortable and pleasant, though he described the Scots as 'manifesting pride, poverty and pianos', a very different picture was painted by the novelist Jerome Weidman.[65] Weidman visited a New York student studying medicine in Edinburgh and supported by his mother, a secretary in New York. This student, Alex Mittelman, was said to have little money and his accommodation was in a 'dirty old tenement with an evil-smelling hallway.....The ceilings were cracked and flaking away and the filthy brown wall-paper in the halls hung down in strips'. Mittelman had a very negative attitude towards his studies and Weidman's published account of Mittelman's views of Americans studying in Edinburgh was deeply resented by the vast majority of Americans studying there. American students were, on the whole, hard-working, industrious and successful but there must have been at least a few 'black sheep' amongst them.

Americans usually contacted the Scottish medical schools before leaving for Europe. Aaron Caplan recalls hearing about Anderson's College from a friend who had been studying for two years in Scotland. He cabled the Dean at Anderson's College and he received a reply saying that he should come to Glasgow with his academic credentials and he did this just prior to the start of the new term in October 1930. Having a science degree he was exempt from taking the courses in the basic sciences but had to take the examinations in these subjects. Herbert Goldberg recalled that the Americans initially had exemption even from the basic science examinations in St. Andrews but that this changed during the 1930's after a trial in which the last group receiving total exemptions were requested to take the examinations, as a guide to the authorities, and they all failed!

When Helen Swiller came to Scotland she arrived without a letter of acceptance and merely had a note of introduction to Dean John Orr of the Medical School of the Royal Colleges in Edinburgh. However, Orr was on holiday and she decided to come to Glasgow. Helen Swiller's parents were not keen for her to study medicine but when she married a prospective medical student their objections disappeared. She and her husband were married on the 28th August 1935 and sailed for Scotland two days later on the Anchor Line 'California'. After the arrangements for the wedding and the travel abroad were made Irving Swiller received an acceptance from an American medical school which he promptly destroyed so that he and his new wife would still be able to study medicine together.

In Glasgow they met Dean Carstairs Douglas at St. Mungo's College who said 'Which God has united let no man tear asunder' and their medical school places were assured. The Swillers proved to be excellent students and they, the only married couple who were both medical students, were vividly recalled decades later by many of their class-mates.

Some students were obviously affected by the War and while some did manage to get back to Scotland to complete their courses others, who were spending the summer vacation at home in 1939, did not manage to return to Scotland. Irwin Kantor, now Professor of Clinical Dermatology at the Mount Sinai School of Medicine and the City University of New York, managed only one year before the War began and did not resume his studies in Edinburgh until 1946 when he returned to the Royal Colleges School of Medicine, which two years later was absorbed by the University of Edinburgh.

Paul Steinlauf was on vacation in Switzerland when the War began. The advice from the American Consul in Scotland was to go home immediately as the U.S. Government would not be responsible for Americans in a country at war. However, he returned to Glasgow to complete his studies. Writing in the *Lister Journal*, the publication of the Glasgow extra-mural medical colleges, Bernard Iskowitz described the negotiations leading to the return of himself and some of his colleagues to Scotland. The first priority was judged to be the 40 final year students stranded in America with passports cancelled and with the help of many public figures the State Department finally relented and allowed the final year students to return.[66] Phil Reisman heard a rumour one summer that a bill was being proposed to prevent American students studying overseas and he spoke to Congressman Fiorello La Guardia who lived in his block and who agreed to take up the matter with Harold Rypins in Albany. A few days later he heard from La Guardia that it was a false alarm.

Even leaving Scotland for the States during the War was hazardous for Americans graduating and wishing to return home. Arthur Beck qualified in July 1940 and in December of that year travelled with some companions to London in the hope of getting on a flight to Lisbon from where he might make the connection to the United States. By the time they reached London the service had been suspended and they were forced to return to Glasgow to await a further opportunity.[67]

The memories that most of the Americans carried back with them from Scotland reflected the sense of achievement in completing their medical studies, but there was far more than that. The Americans were made to feel very welcome in Scotland and enjoyed their stay immensely. They felt that the atmosphere in the various medical schools was much more relaxed than they would have found in the States and they enjoyed a marked degree of camaraderie which existed between all the students. Being foreigners together the Americans co-operated closely with each other and many made friendships which they carried back across the Atlantic and which lasted for the rest of their lives. The financial support enjoyed by St. Andrews University and the Royal College of Surgeons of Edinburgh in particular, is a manifestation both of appreciation about having the opportunity to study and of the friendships which developed among the students there.

The Americans felt that they gained some real advantages by studying in Scotland. They enjoyed the considerable emphasis on clinical judgement and acumen and the continual training in the powers of observation. 'We were taught to look'. This clinical orientation would serve many in good stead in the States. The American medical education was more technical and scientific and the students there were more aware of medical advances. They followed the articles in the medical journals. The pace in Scotland was much more leisurely and Sid Druce remembers that the medical students did not read the journals in Scotland. In fact as a medical student in Edinburgh he did not even know that there *were* medical journals! Druce also commented that therapeutics was more advanced in the States but it did not prove difficult for the returning graduates to adapt to the differences in American medicine. At first Druce had felt inferior to the American students who had studied at home but it was when working as an intern that he appreciated the solid practical training he had received in Edinburgh. In America it was possible to graduate with little or no patient contact and clinical acumen was at a lower level.

There was cut-throat competition in the American medical schools where there was a pre-determined student drop-out rate each year. Consequently students were actively competing against each other for the available places in the following year. By contrast the Scottish experience had been one of friendship and helpfulness and was aided by a collection of charismatic teachers to be found in all the medical centres in Scotland

In Edinburgh Dean John Orr was a particular favourite of the Americans. He had defended their interest loyally and in return the American students repaid him by their high academic achievements. He had treated the Americans generously and with open arms and the Royal Colleges' Medical School was the most popular Scottish medical school for the Americans in the early 1930's. The Americans also recalled many of the most charismatic teachers, such as Johnny Graham in Glasgow, E. B. Jamieson in Edinburgh and Prof. C. Rutherford Dow in Dundee, all of whom taught anatomy.

On returning to the United States the Scottish graduates managed to negotiate the State Board Examinations successfully and there was little difficulty in finding residencies, although places in the more academic hospital programmes were reserved for American graduates. The outbreak of War created a demand for extra physicians which soon ensured that places were found for all the overseas graduates and that some of the difficulties in obtaining the best residences was at an end.

At the height of Dean Rappleye's crusade against the foreign students there had been some problems for foreign graduates in entering residencies and internships and thinly disguised anti-semitism was rife.[68] The returning graduates found that Scottish medicine was held in some respect in the United States although there was a lack of understanding about the nomenclature of the Scottish degrees. In America the basic medical degree is the M.D. and anyone trying to set up in practice with M.B. Ch.B. or LRCP&S, LRFPS on his plate would have run into immediate difficulties. It was not difficult to obtain local M.D.'s (Medical Diplomas) on being licensed to practise in their home states. Paul Steinlauf obtained his 'M.D.' from the New Jersey Board of Medical Examiners which was neither a medical school nor a university.

Table 6:12 Career Choices of Sample of American Graduates in Medicine in Scotland

	No	%
general practice/family practice	44	37.8
general medicine	18	15.7
psychiatry/psychoanalysis	10	8.5
general surgery	9	7.8
dermatology	6	5.2
paediatrics	5	4.2
radiology	5	4.2
obstetrics/gynaecology	5	4.2
anaesthetics	4	3.5
others	10	8.9
Total	116	100.0

source: American Medical Directory, 1982.

Gradually and especially after the War, the Americans who had graduated in Scotland integrated into the American medical scene. Many obtained distinguished academic posts although more than half entered general practice, an unusually high figure in America, which must suggest that opportunities were restricted. Nevertheless it was clear that those with ability had had the opportunity to reach high positions in American medicine (Table 6:12).

The American graduates all look back with fond memories on their studies in Scotland and most said that they would do the same again if the opportunity arose. Some of their sons have returned to study in Scotland, especially in St. Andrews, and the American graduates have helped to fund their old universities and to set up scholarships. Nathaniel Solomon recalled with pride the fund-raising show conducted annually for five years by the American students in Edinburgh on behalf of the Royal Infirmary. It had given them a chance to contribute something to the city and to this day they still feel a debt of gratitude.

REFERENCES

1   Stephen Steinberg, 'How Jewish Quotas Began', *Commentary* Vol. 52, Sept. 1971, p.71
2   *Encyclopaedia Judaica* (Jerusalem 1972) Vol.12, col.1078
3   Stephen Steinberg ibid., p.683
4   Marcia Graham Synott, *The Half-Opened Door:Discrimination and Admissions at Harvard, Yale and Princetown 1900-1970* (Westport 1979) p.XVIII
5   op.cit., p.14
6   Marcia Graham Synott, 'Anti-Semitism and American Universities' in *Anti-Semitism in American History* (University of Illinois 1986) p.236
7   op.cit., p.71

8   'Professional Tendencies Among Jewish Students in Colleges, Universities and Professional Schools', *American Jewish Year Book*, Vol. 22, 1920-1921, pp.383-93, 406-8
9   Nathan Glazer, 'Social Characteristics of American Jews 1654-1954', *American Jewish Year Book*, Vol. 56, 1955, p.24
10 Charles Silbermann, *A Certain People*, (New York 1985) p.53
11 ibid., p.54
12 Marcia Graham Synnott op.cit., p.60
13 Stephen Steinberg op.cit., p.72
14 Marcia Graham Synnott op.cit., p.18
15 Harold S. Wechsler, *The Qualified Student: A History of Selective College Admission in America* (New York 1977) p.134
16 ibid., p.157
17 ibid., p.136
18 ibid., p.162
19 ibid., p.161
20 A. Flexner, 'Medical Education in the United States and Canada' (New York 1910) p.346
21 Saul Jarcho, 'Medical Education in the United States- 1910-1956' *Journal of the Mount Sinai Hospital* Vol. XXXVl no.4, pp.346-7,357
22 ibid., p.344
23 ibid., pp.355-6
24 *Journal of the American Medical Association* Vol. 104, 1935, p.1054
25 J.A.M.A Vol. 104. 1935, p.1055
26 Henry E. Sigerst, 'Trends in Medical Education: A Program for a New Medical School', *Bulletin of the History of Medicine* Vol. 1X (Baltimore 1941) p.181
27 Saul Jarcho op.cit., pp.357-8
28 'Review of the Year 5690', *American Jewish Year Book* Vol. 32, 1930-1931, p.78
29 ibid., p.79
30 'Review of the Year 5691', *American Jewish Year Book* Vol. 33, 1931-1932, pp.55-6
31 Alfred L. Shapiro, 'Racial Discrimination in Medicine' *Jewish Social Studies* Vol. 10, April 1948, p.131
32 ibid., p.106
33 ibid., p.134
34 'Review of the Year 5695', *American Jewish Year Book* Vol. 37, 1935-1936, pp.157-8
35 *Healing and History: Essays for George Rosen* ed. Charles E. Rosenberg, (1979) p.250
36 ibid., p.243
37 Interviews and questionnaires on file.
38 Lawrence Bloomgarden, *A Preliminary Analysis of Discrimination against Jewish Applicants for Admission to Medical School in New York State*, mimeographed and published privately by the American Jewish Committee (1952) pp.18-24
39 Alfred L. Shapiro op.cit., p.103
40 Harold S. Wechsler op.cit., p.169
41 Dan Oren, *Joining the Club: A History of Jews and Yale*, (New Haven, 1985) p.140
42 ibid., p.148
43 ibid., pp.149-55
44 Frank Kingdon, 'Discrimination in Medical Colleges', *The American Mercury* Vol. LX1, No. 262, p.394
45 John Duffy, *The Healers* (Univ. of Illinois 1979) p.290

46   Charles Silbermann op.cit., p.124
47   Charles Reznikoff, 'New Haven: the Jewish Community' *Commentary* Vol. 4, (1947) p.477
48   Jacob A. Goldberg, 'Jews in the Medical Profession' *Jewish Social Studies* Vol. 1, (1939) p.332
49   *Minutes of the General Medical Council for 1930* Vol. LXV11. see appendix X11 (Interim Report of the Colonial and Foreign Students Committee on the Application of American students to study medicine in Great Britain and Ireland) pp.317-8 Memorandum by the Registrar, Norman C. King, on the American Medical Students pp.319-23 Memorandum on Registration of Students, Norman Walker pp.324-7 reports of the Scottish Branch of the General Medical Council pp.455-62
50   *Minutes of the General Medical Council for 1932* Vol. LX1X, p.5
51   Robert Smart, University of St. Andrews Library, personal communication.
52   *Jewish Echo* (Glasgow) gives lists of all Jewish prize and distinction winners.
53   Minutes of the Education Committee and Board of Management of the School of Medicine of the Royal Colleges of Edinburgh
54   Faculty of Medicine application in Senate Minutes, University of Glasgow, 1932-1935
55   Interviews with American graduates of the Scottish medical schools, on file.
56   For information on the Scottish medical schools in the 1930's see : 'Medical Schools in Scotland' *BMJ* 1937(2) pp.476-8
57   'A Plea for Democracy in Medicine' (published by the Physicians Committee Against Discrimination in Medicine) (New York 1946) p.10
58   Jacob A. Goldberg, 'Jews in Medicine', *Medical Economics* March 1940 pp.54-56 In 1937-1938 out of 1298 Americans studying medicine abroad it was estimated that about 90% were Jewish.
59   JAMA Vol. 113, 1939 p.772 'As a result of an inspection made of these schools in November 1938, the New York State Examination Board in January 1939 directed that ......the department no longer issue qualifying certificates to American students seeking admission to these schools'.
60   *Lister Journal*, Vol. 2 no.2, December 1940, p.18
61   'Comments of the Governing Body of the Medical School of the Royal Colleges of Edinburgh on the Goodenough Committee on the Future of Non-University Medical Schools', (privately circulated, Edinburgh)— Library of the Royal College of Surgeons, Edinburgh.
62   *Jewish Echo*, issues of 15, 22 and 29 Nov. and 6 Dec. 1935.
63   *Jewish Echo*, 20 April 1938
64   David Daiches, *Two Worlds: An Edinburgh Jewish Childhood* (Sussex 1971) pp.127-8
65   Jerome Weidman, 'May 27, 1939—Royal Bank of Scotland, St. Andrews Square, Edinburgh, Scotland—$50', *Letter of Credit* (New York 1940) p.111
66   *Lister Journal*, Vol. 2, no.1, p.19
67   *Lister Journal*, Vol. 2, no.2, p.25
68   See, for example, *A Plea for Democracy in Medicine*

SEVEN

European Refugee Physicians in Scotland 1933-1945

During the 1930's and 1940's some hundreds of refugee physicians from Central Europe, who were overwhelmingly of Jewish origin, were given the opportunity to obtain qualifications which could be registered in Britain by taking the examinations of the Scottish Triple Qualification Board.

Refugee physicians began arriving in Britain soon after the Nazi accession to power. The Nazis had moved quickly with their anti-Jewish measures and Jewish doctors were among their first targets. As early as 22nd April 1933 restrictions were placed on the numbers of doctors in National Health Insurance practices and these limits were gradually extended to other medical men.[1,2] By the end of 1933 there had been 60,000 emigrants from Germany, of whom about 80% were Jewish.[3]

Jews had been disproportionately represented in German academic and professional life. They formed barely one per cent of the population but made up 10 per cent of the medical profession and formed one quarter of all German Nobel prize-winners.[4] Deprived of their professional livelihoods on racial grounds in Germany, the refugee physicians sought to enter medical practice in their countries of exile. This was not to be easy as many countries, such as Britain and the United States, had regulations which gave their own nationals certain privileges as far as medical practice was concerned.

The pattern of German policy towards Jewish medical students completing their medical studies had not been definitively laid down by 1934. By March 1934 the admission of non-Aryan medical students was completely restricted.[5] A Jewish medical student, who had completed his studies but had not yet taken his final examinations, had the alternative of trying to take examinations in a country like Italy, with which Britain had reciprocal medical qualification arrangements, or trying to graduate in a university not yet under Nazi control. Thus, it was still possible for Jews to graduate in medicine in Hamburg in 1934.[6] However, those students who had been excluded at an earlier stage of their undergraduate course would have required to start afresh their medical studies abroad and few managed to do this.

By 1936 about 1,800 physicians had left Germany and the largest group, numbering about 650, settled in Palestine. There were about 400 in the United States, where licensing procedures were being progressively tightened even in such 'liberal' states as New York, and about 300 in the United Kingdom.[7] The medical refugees began to arrive in Britain during 1933, although one German Jewish doctor requalified in 1928 after studying at Anderson's College, Glasgow.[8]

The arrival of some medical refugees in Britain during 1933 prompted the Secretary of the British Medical Association, Dr. George Cranston Anderson, to write to the deans of all the British medical schools to remind them that medical qualifications obtained in Britain would enable the doctor to practise in any of the British dominions and colonies.[9] This letter expressed the concern, communicated to the General Medical Council from South Africa, as well as Australia and New Zealand, that it should not be easier, and quicker, to qualify in Britain and move on to these countries than it would have been to qualify in South Africa in the first place.[10] The reply of the General Medical Council had been that the licensing of medical practitioners was solely a matter for the licensing bodies while the GMC concerned itself with the maintenance and improvement of standards.

This reply had also been given to Dr. M. D. Eder, of the newly formed Jewish Medical Emergency Association, who had asked for some easing of the restrictions of the English Conjoint Board.[11] These required foreign physicians to spend two years, instead of one year, from June 1933, in the process of taking British qualifications. This led to Scotland, and not England, becoming the chief destination of refugee physicians.

The same issue of the *BMJ Supplement*, which had contained Dr. G. C. Anderson's letter in September 1933, included a communication from the honorary secretary of the Medical Information Subcommittee of the Jewish Medical and Dental Emergency Association, which was acting in co-operation with the Jewish Refugee Committee. They were anxious to reply to the statement, which had been made at a BMA Council Meeting in July 1933, that over 800 applications had been received in Britain from German doctors. It was pointed out that only 180 foreign doctors had been registered with their committee and that only half of these were seeking British qualifications. A substantial proportion had already been placed in Edinburgh and Glasgow, with smaller numbers in other centres. This concern to allay medical fears over the scale of the immigration was to be a regular concern of both the Jewish bodies and the Home Office, who had to refute wild rumours which were circulating.

The number of refugee doctors entering Britain between 1933 and 1935 was small, and it was made clear to them that obtaining a British qualification gave no guarantee that the practitioner would be able to register for medical practice in Britain. Nevertheless, the spectre that the medical job market would be flooded by an alien influx was being constantly invoked both in sections of the press, such as Lord Beaverbrook's *Daily Express*, and in certain sections of the British medical profession itself.[12]

It was predictable that there would be opposition to the arrival of foreign doctors from the Medical Practitioners' Union, whose General Secretary, Alfred Welply took a consistently anti-alien line. However, the entry of refugee doctors in any number was also opposed strenuously by Lord Dawson of Penn. Dawson, the Royal physician, was also President of the Royal College of Physicians of London, and had espoused progressive policies in regard to the provision of health care. He had been a leading member of the BMA committee set up to formulate plans for the establishment of a Ministry of Health and in 1918 had outlined plans for a comprehensive health service. He had served two terms as President of the BMA and had not been afraid to deal with such controversial issues as birth control and euthanasia.[13]

Speaking at a meeting at the Royal College of Physicians in London in February 1932 Dawson told the members of the various medical licensing bodies present that British medical students should have some protection, and that it should not be unduly easy for foreign practitioners to qualify.[14,15] He said that the admission of foreign doctors would subject British homes to foreign influences and asked why the United Kingdom should be the only country to have such easy terms for the admission of foreign doctors.*

At that meeting it was agreed by all the medical licensing bodies, with the sole exception of the Scottish Triple Qualification Board, to adopt uniform regulations. It would become necessary for the foreign doctor to take an examination in anatomy and physiology and to do two years of clinical work before presentation for the final examinations.

It was Lord Dawson's view, expressed to the Home Secretary, Sir John Gilmour, at a meeting in November 1933, that there might be room in the United Kingdom for a few refugee physicians of special distinction but the 'number that could usefully be absorbed could be counted on the fingers of one hand'.[16] At his meeting with the Home Secretary Lord Dawson said that the view he expressed on the subject of German Jewish doctors had the full and entire support of his Council.[17], who were 'alarmed' by the prospects of these refugee physicians entering the British register. He was sceptical about 'the habit of the Jews to settle in a new civilisation rather than in an old one'. He reiterated the view that people of an established reputation in Germany had 'nothing to teach us and could not be of any advantage to this country'.

Supporting Lord Dawson at the meeting was Sir Holburt Waring, President of the Royal College of Surgeons of England, who accompanied Dawson to the Home Office. Sir Holburt pointed out the numbers of American Jews who were studying medicine in Scotland and then returned to America 'much to the annoyance of the authorities there'. The Home Secretary replied that study and requalification did not automatically confer the right to practise and he noted that it would be impossible to refuse these refugees the opportunity to study and they could not be returned to Germany in view of the situation there. He suggested that the licensing bodies meet again as circumstances had changed since the meeting at the Royal College of Physicians in London in 1932.

In sharp contrast, the Scottish Board continued to allow foreign graduates to take the final examinations after only one year of clinical studies and there was no requirement to take anatomy and physiology examinations. In

---

*The only foreign countries with reciprocity of medical degrees with Britain were Japan and Italy. Mere possession of a Japanese or Italian qualification did not give an automatic entitlement to a place on the GMC Register. (HO45/20516/625466, Public Records Office).

Scotland the foreign graduates would sit the materia medica and pathology examinations on arrival and take the final examinations one year later. It was little wonder that the overwhelming number of refugee physicians requalified in Scotland. Indeed, the Scottish regulations were well known in Germany and refugee doctors sometimes made only the briefest of stops in London, after their arrival in Britain, before making their way to Edinburgh for the examinations there.

After the meeting at the Home Office, Dawson wrote to the Home Secretary asking him to express the opinion that the Scottish Board was the only 'backslider' to the Secretary of State for Scotland who could then communicate this view to the Scottish colleges.[18] Dawson had thought that the Home Secretary had agreed with the English policy that foreign students should commence by taking anatomy and physiology examinations followed by two years of clinical training before the final examinations. In a marginal note to Dawson's letter the Home Secretary recorded that he had not agreed with Dawson's contention but had pointed out to him that the remedy lay with the medical profession. Subsequently, Waring expressed the view that the medical bodies felt they could achieve more by using their own machinery than by going through the Home Office. They intended to continue discussions with the Scottish Board to try to persuade them to bring their regulations into line with those in England. The Scottish Secretary was informed by the Home Secretary about the discussions with the Presidents of the English Royal Colleges, but if any pressure was exerted by this channel, it was singularly ineffective.

Pressure was applied to the Scottish Board by the English medical bodies at a further meeting of the licensing bodies in London in January 1934. The English bodies agreed to tighten the regulations further by increasing the time required for requalification in medicine from two to three years. The Scottish representative present said that it would be useless for him to take a proposal about lengthening the study time back to his Board. It was their view that it was the purpose of the medical licensing bodies to protect the public and not the medical profession.[19] The Scottish Triple Qualification Board remained adamant that the undertakings that they had already given to refugee physicians about requalification regulations should be honoured. They were prepared to stand up to pressure applied on them to try to bring their regulations into line with those in force in England.

Lord Dawson had been expressing the anti-alien sentiments which had been widely current during the 1930's, but it is noteworthy in this context that, during a visit to Nazi Germany in 1936, he was able to sympathise with his German hosts, who included Hitler and von Ribbentropp, about 'Jewish excesses' although he disagreed with the methods then being employed in Germany to deal with the problem.[20] His views had carried some weight within the English medical bodies but he had been unable to influence his Scottish colleagues.

Many reasons can be adduced for the differing Scottish and English attitudes. There was a long Scottish tradition of attracting overseas doctors who would not be expected to practise there. In contrast there was an English expectation that the refugee practitioners would compete for employment with English graduates. It was not unusual for the Scottish medical student body to contain a substantial foreign component based on the twin characteristics of economic good sense allied to humanitarian sentiment. It was thus expected that the refugee practitioners would form yet one more strand in Scotland's export of medical personnel.

The question of accepting some German Jewish medical men was discussed and agreed at a meeting of the Medical Committee of the Glasgow Royal Infirmary on 18th September 1933.[21] It was decided to accept 24 although reservations were expressed about the teaching together of graduates and undergraduates as their education needs differed. It was therefore agreed that the needs of local students should be satisfied before allocations for foreign students were made. The hospital Superintendent, Dr. Grant, took the initiative in this matter after conferring with Dr. John Orr, who was Dean of the Medical School of the Royal Colleges in Edinburgh where most of the remaining Germans were being placed. While there were said to be no places available at the Western Infirmary in Glasgow, the Victoria Infirmary, situated in the south side of Glasgow, had some places for foreign students, and could allocate them once the needs of local students had been met.

This action by Grant and Orr gave hope and encouragement to the refugee physicians, some of whom were in considerable despair at the prospect of being unable to find a medical school which would enable them to continue in their profession. The favourable replies received from Glasgow and Edinburgh by doctors who had written upwards of thirty letters around the country were naturally greeted with great joy.[22] However, not all the refugee doctors were able to proceed immediately to take British qualifications. A number had been so traumatised by their experiences in Germany that they found the prospects of study and examinations an ordeal which would have to be postponed till their health improved.[22] Others worked in a variety of non-medical positions until their services were made available under the wartime medical emergency regulations.[23]

Following the initial acceptance of German Jewish doctors in Edinburgh and Glasgow in 1933-1934, further refugees were accepted for study in the following academic year.[24] In Edinburgh there had been 43 Germans, of whom all but three were medical graduates, at the Medical School of the Royal Colleges in 1933-1934. In June 1934 John Orr reported to a meeting of the Governing Board that he was dealing with applicants who had to receive Home Office permission to study in Britain and that the Germans were being registered as medical students. A meeting of the Glasgow Infirmaries Joint Consultative Committee was called in September 1933, to discuss the situation, the first time the committee had met for more than two and a half years. It was agreed that Germans arriving in Glasgow would be enrolled at St. Mungo's College, the extra-mural school of the Royal Infirmary. St. Mungo's College had been in danger of closing because of the low level of student recruitment but with the influx of students from Germany and America the student roll gradually increased, and the continuation of the College was secured.

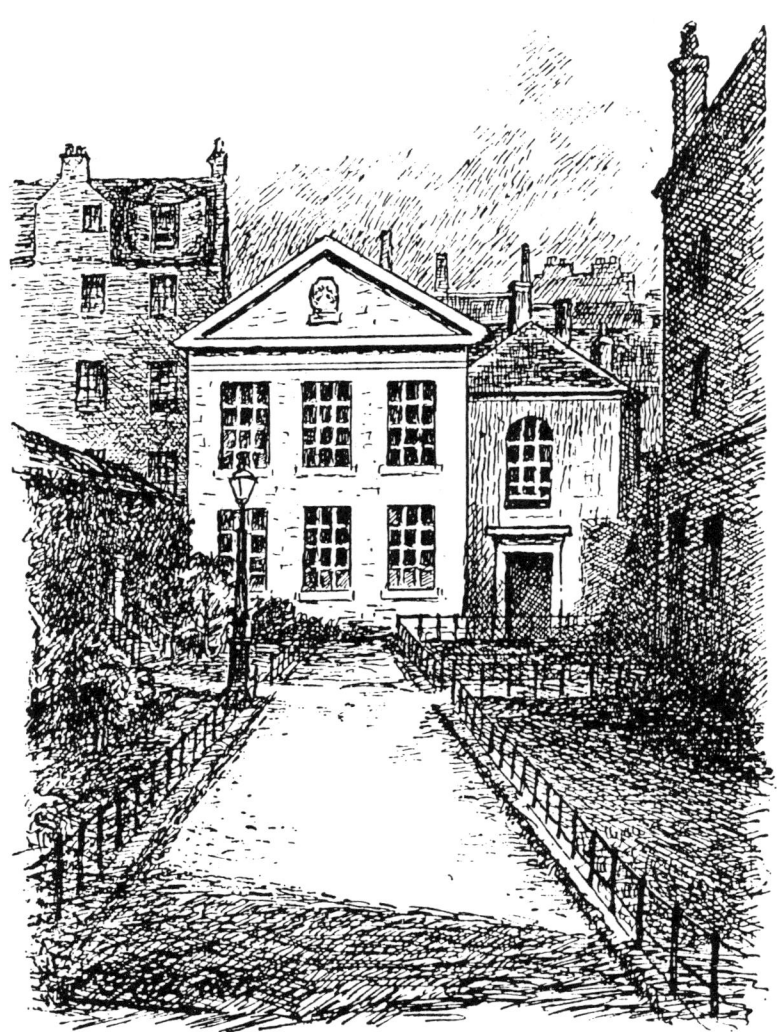
31 The Medical School of the Royal Colleges, Surgeon's Hall, Edinburgh.

As with the American students the position for German medical graduates trying to enter the universities was much more difficult. Unlike the situation in the extra-mural schools, where there was a surplus of teaching places, there was increasing competition for the available space in the medical faculties. In Glasgow, for example, the annual intake of medical students was reduced from 200 to 180 in 1935 as the smaller number was thought to be sufficient for the medical needs of the community, as well as being as much as the hospital teaching facilities could adequately support.[25] As in the discussions over the admission of Americans the priority for admissions was resolved in favour of the interests of local students.

As far as the Germans were concerned, they were seeking short-term clinical and examination facilities and had no interest in undertaking further lengthy undergraduate studies. In this respect the flexibility of the extra-mural colleges suited their needs. Financially too the arrangements at the extra-mural schools were advantageous to the usually impecunious refugees. The fees at most British medical schools ranged from £35 to £50 *per annum* while the examination fees due to the Scottish Triple Qualification Board for all the required subjects, including the Finals was £30.[26]

This led to the further concentration of the overseas medical students in the extra-mural medical schools of Glasgow and Edinburgh. With the needs of the refugee practitioners being met in the extra-mural schools there seemed little need for the universities to allocate any of their scarce places to foreign candidates. By the mid-1930's all applications from students furth of Scotland were being rejected.*

The situation for German refugee physicians was similar in Edinburgh although one student did manage to enter Edinburgh University after leaving his studies in Austria after only one year and after having spent a few months as a research assistant in Cambridge. This student, whose mother was Jewish, was the son of a Professor of Law at Heidelberg and his entry to the Medical Faculty in 1934 was regarded by the Dean as Edinburgh's 'gift' to Heidelberg University on the occasion of its 400th anniversary![27]

This concentration of overseas students in the extra-mural medical schools created some friction between the universities and the extra-mural schools over the usage of shared facilities. The University of Glasgow expressed its concern over the number of alien students receiving tuition in the Pathology Department of the Glasgow Royal Infirmary, as the University had certain rights for its students under regulations dating back some twenty years. However, the managers of the Royal Infirmary rejected this criticism and insisted that the running of the Pathology Department should remain in their hands.[28]

Orr had little difficulty persuading his colleagues in the Edinburgh extra-mural college that he was not interpreting the regulations too widely both by the admission of significant numbers of refugee doctors and by giving them

---

*Minutes of the Senate, University of Glasgow for 1934 show that there were over 100 applications from German doctors.

exemption from language testing on account of their relative fluency in the English language. He was given permission, with little dissension, to continue his liberal admission policy as he had been able to show that there was surplus teaching capacity at the Edinburgh Royal Infirmary.[29] His policy was endorsed at a subsequent meeting of the Governing Board where there was only one dissenting voice out of fifteen members.

Even though the Scottish regulations permitted successful candidates to complete their requalification in one year there were cases in which the progress was even more rapid. A former Professor of Internal Medicine at the University of Berlin lived for a time in both Edinburgh and Glasgow while he prepared to take the examinations of the Triple Qualification Board. He sat his finals after only nine months, after special permission, but failed the examinations! In his case the Home Office also agreed to make an exception in not requiring him to make an undertaking to leave the country after qualifying, as was required with some others.[30]

While some of the examiners encountered by the refugees proved to be difficult, few of the refugee doctors reported problems with the actual conduct of written papers or oral examinations. Many of the examiners were extremely tolerant towards their highly qualified candidates, some of whom had international medical reputations, and orals were conducted in a friendly and social manner.[31,32]

Orr must also have been very patient with the refugee doctors. One had arrived too late for enrolment but Orr was eventually convinced of the candidate's determination after the doctor had made repeated visits to his office. This doctor managed to solve his English language problems by reading the *The Scotsman* and by frequent visits to the Leith Repertory Theatre as well as by talking to as many people as possible.[33] The wife of one of the refugee doctors described the course her husband had taken as 'rather a farce'. The teachers in the Faculty, she recalled, could not help but recognise his superior knowledge and exempted him from lectures and classes.[34]

Some of the German refugees reported feeling that they were second-class citizens within the extra-mural colleges but this feeling, shared by some of the Americans, may have reflected the general status of these colleges within the medical framework of Edinburgh and Glasgow. In any case the classes were helpful for those making their first efforts to adapt to British medicine.

About half of those refugees taking the Triple Qualification had done so by 1936 and numbers fell gradually over the next few years, although they still made up more than 10% of the new licentiates of the Scottish colleges until 1941, when the wartime emergency regulations were introduced (Table 7:1). This indicates that most of the German refugees who took the Scottish qualifications arrived in Britain in the early years of the Nazi persecution, and the numbers of those taking the examinations fell as the number of practitioners entering the country dropped both under pressure from the medical organisations and with the increasing difficulties in leaving Germany. However, even the total numbers of those becoming Scottish licentiates did not amount to 1% of the British medical profession.

Some of the initial problems of adapting to British medicine were ameli-

Table 7:1 Refugee Doctors Obtaining Scottish Triple Qualification

	No. of Refugees	Total No of Licentiates	% Refugees
1934	75	148	50.7
1935	83	203	40.9
1936	25	159	15.7
1937	43	199	21.6
1938	37	204	18.2
1939	31	237	13.1
1940	20	221	9.0
1941	16	138	11.6
1942	2	125	1.6
1943	6	103	5.8
1944	7	117	6.0
1945	4	132	3.0
TOTAL	352	1986	17.7

source: Matriculation Albums of the Scottish Triple Qualification Board.

orated by the assistance of various welcoming organisations. On the Jewish side there were groups like the Jewish Refugees Committee and the Jewish Medical and Dental Emergency Association. Other religious groups, such as the Quakers, were also active in refugee aid and in arranging for resettlement in Britain.[35] Converted Jews also had their own network of support and others were able to build on relationships which they had built up in Britain over the years.[36] For example, those associated with Kurt Hahn, founder of Gordonstoun School, had the benefit of personal contacts with many people throughout Britain whom they had previously met through Hahn's earlier educational activities.[37]

In British academic circles the response was the founding of the Academic Assistance Council (AAC) which arose out of the expressions of creative sympathy within the British universities.[38] The Council rendered singular service to refugees with a scientific or academic background. Later, as the Society for the Protection of Science and Learning (SPSL), it co-operated with the Jewish organisations as it acknowledged that as not all the refugees were Jewish then not all the burden of relief should fall on the Jewish community. At times the Jewish organisations were under such pressure from the volume of relief services required that they were grateful that other organisations and agencies were also involved.

The AAC was founded in May 1933 responding to Hitler's attacks on free learning in Germany. Later the geographical scope of the Council widened as applications came in from other countries, but its limitation to academic personnel was strictly enforced. Thus there were many anguished pleas for help from those whose academic criteria did not meet the required standards. Sir William Beveridge, the Secretary of the Council, and one of its prime movers, wrote that he wished that they had established more effective co-operation with a body which could have helped those in the learned professions. Nevertheless, among the academic refugees were a considerable number with medical qualifications.

The AAC Council faced continual financial problems but its transformation into the SPSL in December 1935 heralded a fresh determination to develop activities further.[39]* It was also intended to build up an Academic Assistance Fund to award research fellowships tenable in the British universities for the most distinguished of the refugee scholars. Placements were carried out on an individual basis as it was soon learned that group placements were rarely successful. An Academic Assistance Committee was founded in Glasgow in 1935 with donations of £345 to found a scholarship which was first held by a photochemist. Research medical scientists who were not likely to find such scholarships easy to obtain were advised rather to take the Scottish Triple Qualification.[40]

The University and hospitals also conducted negotiations with a number of medical scientists although a number of those offered places in Glasgow were able to take up options elsewhere. In addition to its funding from the academic world the SPSL had some financial support from such Jewish organisations as the Central British Fund for German Jewry and the Council of German Jewry. The SPSL retained complete discretion in its expenditure as there was every confidence that the work of the Society would be conducted fairly and correctly.

A proportion of the refugees were political rather than religious and some of those labelled as Jews by the Nazis were not 'confessionally Jewish'. Some, in fact, did not recognise themselves as being Jewish and others would not have been considered as Jews by the Orthodox authorities. About 70% of those on the SPSL lists were estimated to be Jewish, and as many of the Jewish refugees went directly to Jewish groups, the overall proportion of Jews among the refugees, including medical refugees, would thus have been much higher than 70%.

The Jewish Professional Committee parallelled the work of the SPSL and the Jewish Refugees Committee gave individual care to the stream of refugees whose abilities covered a wide range of commerical and professional activities. The placement of German doctors caused great difficulty and even the greatest names in German medicine were not accommodated easily. An Aberdeen professor described the attitude of his Senate as 'friendly helplessness' and noted that the Principal was keen on international problems but that there were 'damnably few posts for which such people are suitable'.[40]

Doctors proved to be harder to place than academics whose fields of study had a more international character. It was not easy for British doctors to admit a group of doctors who were perceived to be a nuisance or even a threat to their own medical incomes. Initially some doctors had to find

---

*By 1938 the SPSL register had 1,400 names from Germany, 418 from Austria and 140 from Italy.

employment outside medicine altogether. It was not uncommon for refugee doctors to take what work they could get in teaching and nursing and many women doctors were first employed as domestics.[41] While the work of integrating the academics was seen as part of the great British tradition of welcoming refugees from persecution there was more professional jealousy involved in the admission of both doctors and lawyers.

British opposition to the admission of German doctors was welcomed in the Nazi press and headlines like 'Morally Unsuited: English Doctors Object to Jewish Practitioners' helped them to suggest that anti-semitism was a widely shared international force.[42] It was left to the *Lancet* to ask whether Britain had all the medical care it wanted in every part of the country or even all the medical care it was prepared to pay for.[43] The *Daily Express* and other popular papers carried anti-alien agitation and there were even suggestions that alien psychoanalysts were exerting a malevolent influence on their British patients.[42]

The cautious welcome given to the refugees in 1933 and 1934 gradually changed over the following years. The numbers attempting requalification remained small and some of the doctors were only a few years off retiral age. Not all the doctors who managed to requalify would automatically be placed on the medical register, and it was expected that a number would move on to other countries such as the United States. Sir Samuel Hoare, later Lord Templewood, was asked, as Home Secretary, in 1937 how many alien doctors had been admitted in the past two years. He answered that there had been 183 in this category and that Home Office policy remained that of closely restricting the entry of foreign doctors.[44] The test for admission was whether an applicant was likely to be an asset to the United Kingdom. Those with an international medical or scientific reputation or who required political asylum, would have a special claim but the 'rank and file' of medical men would be considered unsuitable.

In July 1938 Hoare stated in Parliament that while traditional hospitality would be extended to refugees, the individuals would have to be screened carefully.[45] He acknowledged that some of the Austrian practitioners now under threat following the Anschluss could make a useful contribution to British medicine and he believed that refuge could be afforded to a number of practitioners without flooding the country with practitioners who were not required. Hoare met with representatives of the British Medical Association, the Royal Colleges, London University and the Society of Apothecaries to discuss the admission of some Austrian doctors. The Home Secretary was aware that a humanitarian gesture was called for and his sympathies were with the refugees.[46] It was the opposition of the medical profession, in particular the British Medical Association under pressure from the Medical Practitioners' Union, which limited the numbers admitted to fifty.[47] A selection committee was then set up.

The Medical Practitioners' Union were the bitterest opponents of the admission of refugees. They had shown some sympathy with the problem before 1936 but the policy became one of outright hostility after Dr. Maurice Bayly assumed leadership.[48] In 1938 the MPU said that it would not agree to any refugees being admitted no matter how desperate their plight, and this attitude undoubtedly influenced the BMA response to Hoare's proposal to admit 500 Austrian doctors. The MPU was also prepared to exploit the potential for antisemitism amongst British practitioners by pointing out the different habits in conducting medical practice which the refugees would introduce. This, for example, affected the continental practice of patients expecting direct access to private medical practitioners, instead of the British practice where the introduction to the specialist was made by the general practitioner.

Alfred Welply, General Secretary of the MPU, wrote to British doctors in July 1938 urging them to protest to their M.P.'s at the 'threatened invasion' by foreign doctors. In a further letter in September 1938 Welply ridiculed the BMA and pointed out that the limitation placed on the Austrian doctors to 50, instead of the proposed 500, had come about as a result of MPU's public protests which had been taken up in the popular press.*

The whole international refugee problem was discussed at Evian in 1938 and the British Government took the view there that while they could not specify figures they would be prepared to 'adopt a liberal attitude in the matter of admissions'.[49] Britain was particularly worried about the potential exodus of refugees from Danzig in 1938 because there were certain British obligations there under the League of Nations. The difficulty about doing anything to help was highlighted when Lord Halifax felt it necessary to intercede with the Home Office to secure the admission to Britain of 3 Danzig doctors.[50] The Home Secretary was prepared to accede to the request although he was aware that even this gesture would be opposed by the BMA. A further 50 doctors were admitted after the fall of Prague.

In fact the only form of international relief which would have afforded the refugees the assistance which they required was the widespread lowering of immigration barriers. Most nations were prepared to do no more than to suggest this course of action for their neighbours.

The admission of the doctors from Austria and Czechoslovakia prompted the reduction of the period of clinical study required by the English Conjoint Board from three to two years but this still meant that the requirements were shorter in Scotland. Thus the flow of practitioners northwards to take their final medical examinations in Edinburgh continued. The numbers had been falling after 1937 as doctors postponed their chances of re-entering the medical profession and took up non-medical posts instead. However, it should still be remembered that many refugee doctors were continuing to sit for the Triple Qualification. Not all were studying in Scotland, as some other medical schools, such as in Manchester, were helping candidates prepare for the Scottish examinations. The large majority of refugees taking the Triple Qualification in 1934 and 1935 had studied in Scotland but from 1936 an increasing number were studying in London, Manchester, Birmingham and Cardiff. Nevertheless, the number studying in Glasgow and Edinburgh remained

---

* Correspondence file of Angus MacNiven on the refugee psychiatrists, Gartnavel Royal Hospital, Greater Glasgow Health Board Archives.

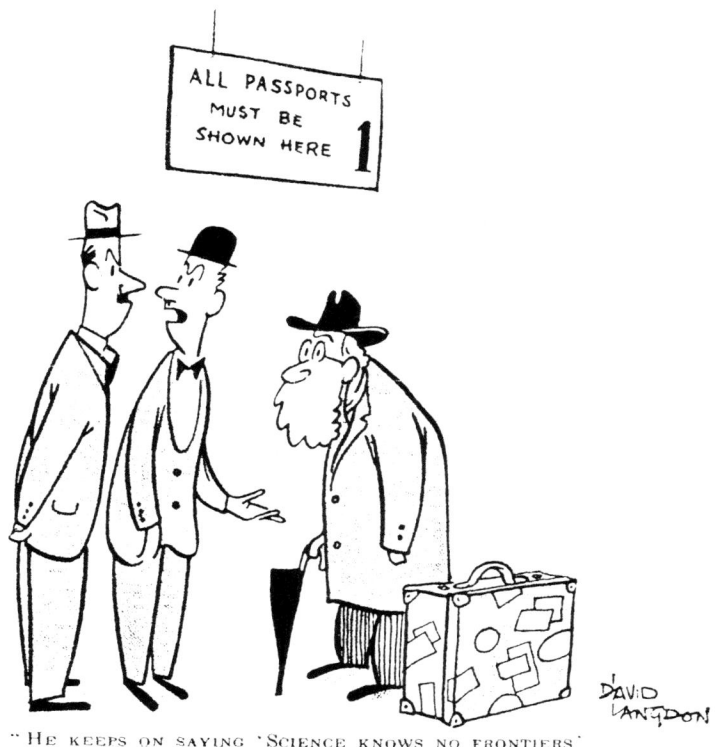

"He keeps on saying 'Science knows no frontiers'—and he hasn't a passport."

32 *Punch* cartoon of August 1938 graphically illustrates the problems faced by refugee scientists and physicians.

important and outnumbered any of the other British medical centres outside London (Table 7:2).

While the numbers using the facilities of the extra-mural medical schools continued, the situation in Scottish universities was quite different. In June 1938 Edinburgh University Medical Faculty stated that they were in general sympathy with 'the many Austrian students whose racial origins or political sympathies had caused them to be placed in a most unfortunate position' but they were mindful of the current climate of opinion in Britain and felt that it would be unwise to provide special facilities for the admission of foreign students. Later in the year, however, the University did agree to admit 3 Czech doctors on a request from Sir Robert Hutchison, Chairman of the Home Office Advisory Committee. In December 1938 they agreed to take one of the Austrians, with exemption from university fees, after receiving another letter from Sir Robert Hutchison, this time in his capacity as Chairman of the Refugee Selection Committee.

At the University of Glasgow the Medical Faculty also decided in June 1938 not to undertake the free education of one Austrian Jewish student. In fact

Table 7:2   Place of Study of German Licentiates

	Glasgow	Edinburgh	London	Others	Total
1934	18	37	13	7	75
1935	28	17	25	13	83
1936	4	5	14	2	25
1937	10	7	22	4	43
1938	7	10	16	4	37
1939	1	8	18	4	31
1940	3	3	12	2	20
1941	3	5	5	3	16
TOTAL	74	92	125	39	330

source: Matriculation Album of the Triple Qualification Board

the Glasgow attitude at this time to the refugees appears to have been unfriendly. Sir Hector Hetherington was unwilling to chair a fund-raising meeting or to sign a petition on behalf of the refugees because of his official position as Principal of the University.[51] Sir Hector had been actively campaigning for an end to the extra-mural medical schools which he felt were of benefit only to the freelance teachers who drew their income from the students and paid only a token charge for the facilities they enjoyed.[52] Sir Hector was concerned at the very considerable numbers of overseas students in the extra-mural schools, which he felt led to the exclusion of qualified British students from the available places. However, his reference to 'less eligible aliens in less reputable institutions' was intended only to imply criticism of Anderson's and St. Mungo's Colleges and not any antagonism to Jews *per se* as eligible local Jews continued to be admitted to the university.[53]

In Aberdeen, no German doctors or medical students were admitted in 1933 as priority was being given to local candidates.[54] However, Hans Kosterlitz was admitted as a research student in physiology in 1933 and permitted to take clinics to qualify for the Triple Qualification in 1938. Kosterlitz subsequently had a distinguished academic career in Aberdeen, becoming Professor of Pharmacology in 1968. In 1938 the Senate agreed to take an Austrian medical student without fees and in 1939 3 German doctors were admitted to research projects.[54]

Thus the portal of entry into British medicine for the refugees remained substantially through the Scottish Triple Qualification; even Kosterlitz, a researcher in a university department found this the easiest route to a British qualification. The examinations of the Scottish Triple Qualification Board were being taken either after study in the extra-mural schools or at an approved hospital, usually in London but also at some other British centres.

Thus the traditional liberal voice of the Scottish universities was muted during the response to the influx of refugee physicians. The universities made a number of useful gestures but they could not compete with the practical facilities offered by the extra-mural schools. The universities were undoubtedly concerned about the needs of local students and they were aware that the needs of the foreign students were being met not just in the lecture theatres of the extra-mural schools but in the very hospital teaching facilities that the universities and colleges shared.

There was a definite antagonism between the universities and the extra-mural medical schools and the fact that the extra-mural schools could pursue an independent policy while dependent on many of the teaching facilities attached to the universities, increased their vulnerability. Thus the universities were able to use the very attraction of the foreign students to these schools as a prime reason for the need to abolish them.

The Scottish extra-mural colleges were not alone in the medical profession in expressing their sympathy for the German doctors. Concern was being expressed during 1938 in the correspondence columns of the *Lancet*. Fears had been expressed that the refugee physicians had a natural advantage in that the British public looked on the continentals as being in a 'higher category'. There were worries about competition and about the number of doctors setting up their plates in Harley Street. Samson Wright, the distinguished physiologist who was active in Jewish refugee relief, was constrained to reply that only 187 German doctors had been licensed since 1933 in a profession which numbered over 50,000.[55] However, it was acknowledged that this figure did not include the greater number of doctors who hoped to get on the Medical Register. It was also appreciated that while it was worthwhile to express the hope that surplus European doctors were needed in the under-doctored areas of the world it was these areas which did not have the resources to employ such personnel.

As against these concerns the editorial policy of the *Lancet* expressed the contrary viewpoint in February 1939 entitled 'As Others See Us'.[56] It suggested that the restrictive position of the medical bodies had done the profession no good and said that 'if we become infected with national exclusiveness' the medical ideals of science and service could be lost. It would be recognised by an outsider that the interests of the community as a whole do not always coincide with those of the sections of which it is composed. To make doctors do other work, or no work at all, would be a great human waste. The appeal of those like Welply to sectional self-interest was an unpleasant development in medical politics and the *Lancet* was concerned that medicine and humanity which had previously been considered as inseparable concepts were no longer being regarded in this light. It was left to William Temple, Archbishop of York and President of the SPSL to say that what was being done for the desperate needs of the refugees would be 'preparing a way for the return of civilised life and hopes among men'.[56]

In fact there were activities being carried out on a local level to help refugee practitioners which helped to keep alive this very concept of medicine and humanity. With the increasing numbers of Jewish doctors coming out of Austria there were particular problems facing the psychiatrists and psychoanalysts in Britain where the field had been less well developed than it was in Vienna, the centre of pyschoanalysis. In May 1938 the Secretary of the

Institute of Psychoanalysis, Dr. Edward Glover wrote to Dr. Angus MacNiven, Physician Superintendent at Glasgow's Gartnavel Royal Hospital, to enlist his support in placing refugee psychiatrists in Glasgow. On an international level this activity was being conducted by Dr. Ernest Jones as President of the International Psychoanalytical Association.[57]

Through 1938 and 1939 MacNiven attempted to find places for Austrian psychiatrists as clinical assistants, mental nurses or as clinical clerks. However the problems of obtaining work permits were often unsurmountable even when arrangements for financing of posts had been found. MacNiven was given permission by the BMA to take on a refugee physician as an unpaid Clinical Clerk on condition that no offical documents were signed and though the General Board of Control at the Scottish Office gave permission this arrangement was vetoed by the Home Office. MacNiven was unable to find a place in Glasgow for Erwin Stengel whom Glover described as a psychiatrist of 'unusually brilliant attainments'.

Nevertheless despite these difficulties Gartnavel Royal included on its staff a number of psychiatrists on varying clinical attachments. There were several women refugee practitioners working as psychiatric nurses as well as a female refugee psychiatrist holding a clinical attachment. In addition, the staff had the services of Karl Abenheimer, a former lawyer and judge in Mannheim, who had trained in analytical techniques with Jung in Vienna and who was involved with MacNiven and David Yellowlees from 1936 in the running of the Lansdowne Clinic in Glasgow, on the lines of the Tavistock Clinic in London. MacNiven referred patients to Abenheimer who maintained a private practice outside his work at Gartnavel and his work for the Lansdowne Clinic which was supported by charitable donations. At the time there was thought to be little scope for private practitioners in psychoanalysis and psychotherapy as MacNiven noted that well-to-do patients suffering from psychoneuroses were rarely referred to psychiatrists.

At Crichton Royal too good use was made of refugee psychiatric expertise. In 1937 Dr. Peter K. McGowan was appointed Physician Superintendent and although he was a practitioner with a traditionalist background he was receptive to the ideas of developing research and in bringing to Crichton Royal figures of distinction in the psychiatric world. The Board agreed with this policy and in June 1939 Dr. Willy Mayer-Gross was appointed Director of Clinical Research.[58] Mayer-Gross had been Associate Professor at the University of Heidelberg but seeing as early as 1932 that there would be no future in Germany for those with Jewish origins he came to Britain where a Rockefeller Foundation scholarship provided the opportunity to take the position of Research Fellow at the Maudsley Hospital.[59] He held this post until taking the Triple Qualification in 1939 and entering his new post in Dumfries where he set up an Insulin Unit for the treatment of schizophrenia but also built up laboratory resources and mounted an intensive mental health survey in the area.[60] The combined reputations of Mayer-Gross and McGowan enabled the attraction of a stream of distinguished young psychiatrists to Crichton Royal. These included other refugee psychiatrists who served as assistant physicians and house physicians and the clinical assistants also had

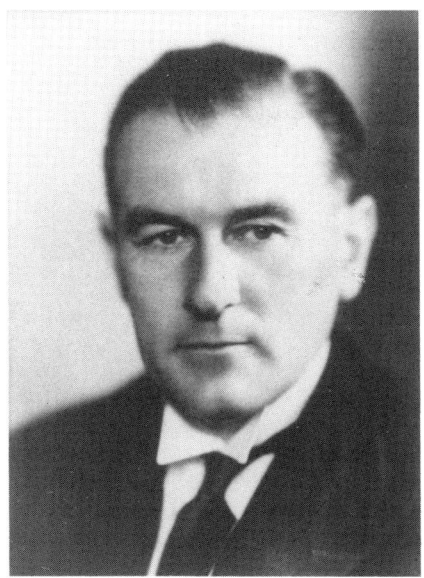

33 Peter McGowan, Medical Superintendent of Crichton Royal, Dumfries.

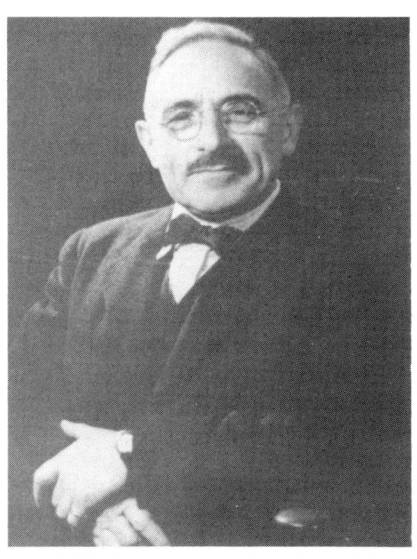

34 Willi Meyer-Gross, Director of Clinical Research, Crichton Royal, Dumfries.

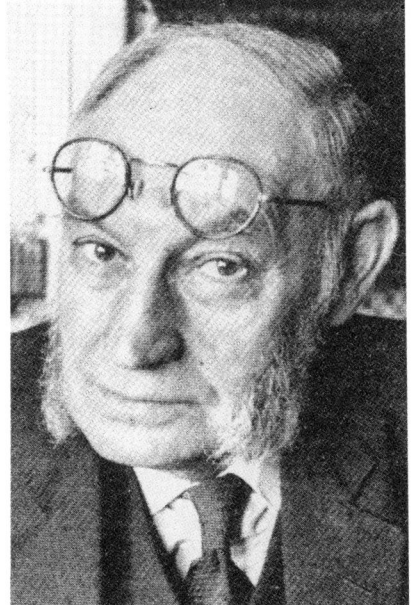

35 Angus MacNiven, Medical Superintendent of Gartnavel Royal, Glasgow.

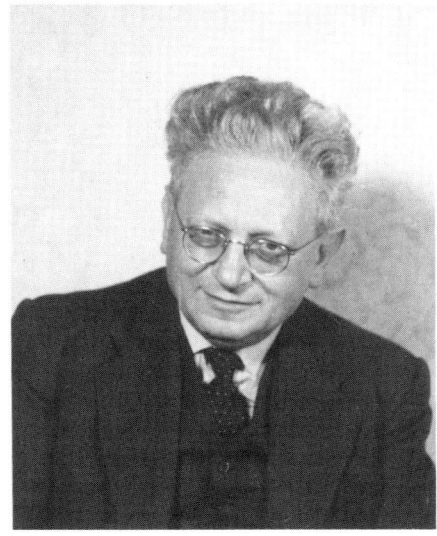

36 Karl Abenheimer, jurist and pioneer of psychoanalysis in Scotland.

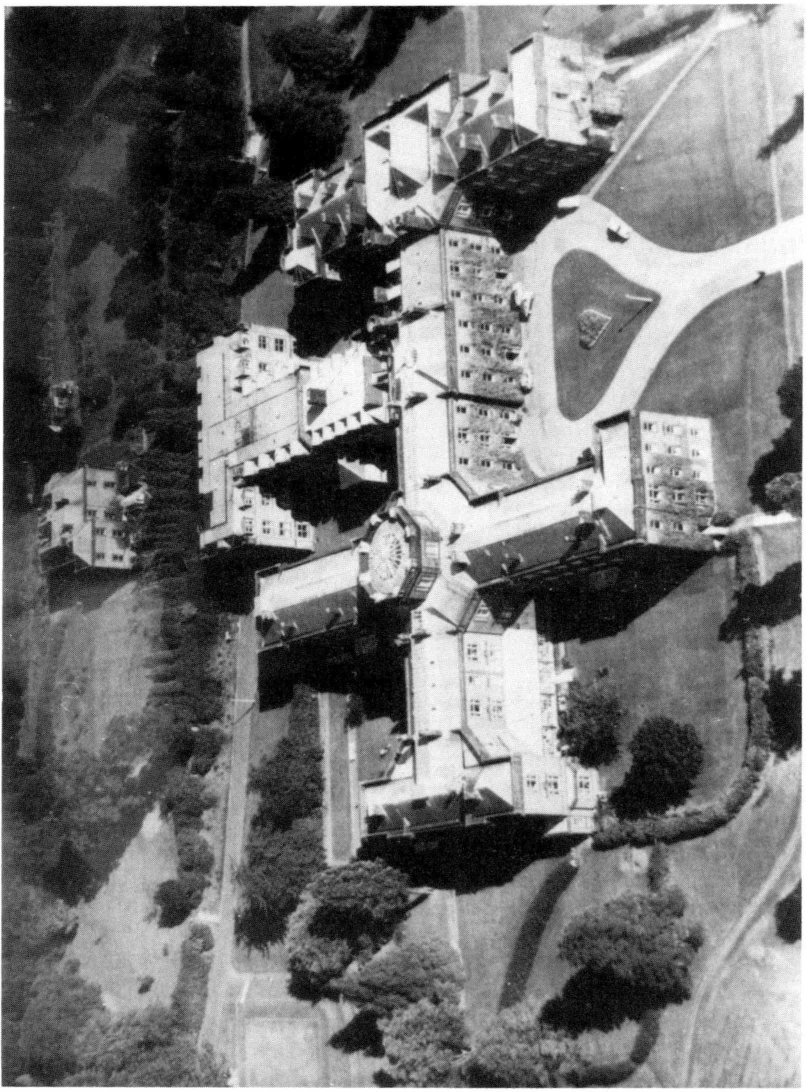

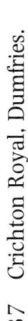

37 Crichton Royal, Dumfries.

an international flavour and included a number of the Americans who were completing their medical studies in wartime Scotland.

In Edinburgh too, refugee psychiatrists were integrated into the hospital services. Sir David Henderson's staff at the Royal Edinburgh Hospital contained a number of refugee psychiatrists who were involved in psychotherapy and psychiatric research. One of the first was Herbert Rosenfeld who arrived in Edinburgh in 1935 and later achieved an international reputation for his work on psychotic states. Erwin Stengel, who had been interned in 1940, was research fellow at the Royal Edinburgh Hospital from 1942 until he took up the post of Senior Psychiatrist at Crichton Royal, which he held for three years. During this time Stengel took the Triple Qualification in 1944. He later became Professor of Psychiatry in Sheffield in 1956.

Felix Post, who later had a distinguished career at the Maudsley Institute of Psychiatry specialising in the psychiatry of old age, spent three years at the Royal Edinburgh Hospital before joining the RAMC in 1945.

Another pyschoanalyst who made a considerable contribution to the Scottish scene was William Kraemer who had left Nazi Germany in 1933 and avoided the need for British qualifications by taking his medical degree in Siena in Italy. Kraemer undertook a Jungian analytical training and was involved in the innovative Freud-Jung group in the early 1960's when the two psychoanalytical schools had little communication between each other. Kraemer was the main colleague in 1939 of Winifred Rushforth as the founder of the Davidson Clinic in Edinburgh. The clinic specialised in group, occupational and child therapy as well as in analysis and it ran without outside support until closed by the National Health Service in 1964. Kraemer was also co-founder of the Marriage Guidance Council of Scotland.

In addition to the refugee contribution to the delivery of medical care, especially in the field of psychiatry, the onset of war gave further scope for the utilisation of the skills of all those medical refugees who found themselves in Britain. To augment the specialist pool the newly formed Emergency Medical Services (EMS) could call on some 500 refugee practitioners.[61] Under Defence Regulation 32B the General Medical Council was empowered to give temporary registration to physicians who had qualified in such countries as Germany, Italy, Poland and Czechoslovakia. Regulations were clarified with an Order in Council in November 1941 which made clear that doctors from the various countries would be placed on the Register and would be eligible for civilian service.[62]

In addition to the 500 doctors who entered the EMS the remaining 800 refugee doctors, who had not yet obtained British qualifications, were also placed on the Register.[63] Despite this a number of doctors still came to Edinburgh to take the Triple Qualification, possibly because they felt that the new war regulations might prove to be temporary. However, the doctors who were temporarily registered during the war were placed on the permanent Register following the passage of the Medical Practitioners and Pharmacists Act of 1947.

With the onset of war the British authorities were worried about leaving potentially harmful alien fugitives at liberty and an indiscriminate internment system was introduced which separated people from other members of their family and often interred genuine refugees together with Nazi sympathisers.[64] The internment policy was described as 'an obscurantist act' by Sir Samuel Hoare[65] and caused much frustration and some resentment among the internees. If any benefit arose from the internment policy the identification of Nazi sympathisers was aided and some refugees who were sent on to Australia and Canada from internment found employment easier there than it would have been in Britain.[66]

During the period of internment Edinburgh became a restricted area and it was easier to obtain employment in Glasgow. One pathologist obtained employment in Glasgow after leaving internment at Huyton, near Liverpool, thanks to contacts that Professor Provan Cathcart had with Professor Durig and his department in Vienna.[67] Others fared less well. One occupational health specialist was sent on to Canada from internment on the Isle of Man and had a 'tough time' on return trying to revise for the final examinations which he passed in Edinburgh in 1941.[68]

As the war progressed the number of refugee doctors in employment increased. In May 1941 less than 10% were in employment, the figure of 700 unemployed alien practitioners being given in April 1941. This number fell slowly during the rest of 1941 and by the beginning of 1942 the number in employment had risen to 64%.[69] There was still some antipathy to the employment of alien doctors but by the end of the war their outstanding contribution to the British war effort was widely acknowledged.

None of this impressed the MPU. Even at the end of the war they maintained their hostility to alien doctors and were prepared to send all the alien doctors 'home'. They even frowned on a scheme to send British medical students to help the work of rehabilitating concentration camp survivors at Belsen.[69] Their anti-alien policy was not changed until 1947.

Despite the activities of the MPU and others who were hostile to the medical refugees the majority of the Germans had pleasant memories of their stay in Scotland, despite the problems with the language and the strain on older doctors of a return to medical studies. For some, however, the definite objective of the Scottish qualifications was a simpler goal than the struggle for a suitable job after leaving Glasgow or Edinburgh.[70] The atmosphere was easier in 1933 and 1934 when there was considerable sympathy for the plight of the refugees. As war approached there was increase in 'spy fever' and all foreigners, no matter their sympathies, were treated with suspicion. In 1933 it had been easier to enter Britain as no visa was required if evidence of financial support could be provided.

The refugees formed their own social circles. In Glasgow a number found comfort in the meetings of Glasgow Zionists and in the support of Dr. Lewis Rifkind, a Glasgow practitioner, who displayed an early profound understanding of the German Jews and their plights.[71] One anaesthetist who, although a refugee from Germany, was actually a British subject as his father had been born in London, became the subject of a policy enquiry after rumours that he was a spy during the time he spent in Glasgow moving among Central European refugees.[72]

Other refugees found the climate in Edinburgh congenial. Desider Engel, a surgeon of some repute, obtained exemption from classes and divided his time in Edinburgh, with financial support from the Rockefeller Foundation, between the neuro-surgical department of Norman Dott and the surgical research laboratory of Sir David Wilkie.[73] Engel, like many of his colleagues, recalled Wilkie as an outstanding lecturer, surgeon and researcher, and the memories of Wilkie and of Sir John Fraser confirm the refugees' predelicition for surgical teaching. Engel enjoyed his stay in Edinburgh and was able to prepare for his surgical fellowship examinations in Edinburgh, and at the same time see something of Scotland, by undertaking surgical locums in Kirkwall, in Orkney, and on the island of Benbecula in the Outer Hebrides.

The Scottish universities had been unable or unwilling to accommodate many of the German or Austrian refugees but the war years in Edinburgh saw one further remarkable story in the role of Scotland in international medical education. A Polish School of Medicine was established at the University of Edinburgh in February, 1941.[74] This was set up at a time when Poland was under foreign occupation and was seen initially as a contribution to building up Polish medicine after the war, although few of its graduates chose to return there. The Polish Army units in Scotland had a surplus of medical staff with many specialists who lectured in their subjects while such chairs as could not be filled by Poles were filled by Professors from the University of Edinburgh. To facilitate training the Edinburgh City Council designated part of the Western General Hospital with 130 beds as the Paderewski Hospital. The first M.B. Ch.B. degrees were conferred in December 1941 and the number of graduates increased to 33 in 1943. At the end of the war there were no further admissions to the Polish School of Medicine and to enable those students who first matriculated in 1944-45 to complete their studies it was agreed to close the School in 1949.

During the nine sessions there were 228 graduates from the Polish School of Medicine and some 19 obtained the postgraduate degree of M.D. A further 33 students graduated at other British universities after transferring in 1946 and there were students who discontinued their studies at various stages of their undergraduate careers.

The Jewish community in pre-war Poland had been proportionately the largest in the world outside of Palestine. The 3,350,000 Jews in Poland in September 1939 made up over 10% of the total Polish population and in the great urban centres such as Warsaw, Lodz and Bialystok the Jewish proportion approached one third. There were restrictive anti-Jewish measures in the Polish universities and many Polish Jews studied abroad. In 1928-9 only 10% of Jewish university students in Poland were studying medicine and in 1932-3 there were 900 Polish Jews studying in Prague.[75] Nevertheless, the Jews made up nearly one fifth of Poland's university students in 1929-30. This was just under twice their proportion in the general population though less than their proportion in the urban centres. Between 1929 and 1938 the Jewish percentage studying medicine fell by almost half.[76]

It would be expected that any group of Polish subjects during the war would include a number of Jews. The Polish School of Medicine in Edinburgh included a few Jews on the Faculty; Jewish students also made up about 9% of the total graduation, up to 1949, and just under 5% of the graduates up to the end of 1945. Thus the Polish School of Medicine provided an opportunity for a number of Polish Jews to complete their medical studies in Scotland.

After the war the refugee practitioners gradually dispersed all over Britain and some emigrated. By 1986 a little more than half of the survivors were in the London area, with about 10% still in Scotland, mostly in Glasgow and Edinburgh. Many of the refugees found it difficult to enter their former specialities in Britain and the largest group entered general practice but with many in internal medicine, psychiatry and the surgical specialities (Table 7:3).

A number continued their private practices in Harley Street, some serving purely refugee clientele. Those with international reputations maintained worldwide medical contacts and some like the allergist Herbert Herxheimer and Willy Mayer-Gross were invited to return to Germany

Although the greatest number of the refugees were to be found in general practice their specialist skills were of immense value to Aneurin Bevan in finding the specialists he needed to augment the relatively low numbers of British consultants in the setting up of the National Health Service.[77] The case for giving the refugees permanent status, already strong on ethical and humanitarian grounds, became incontestable when considered against the prospective specialist shortage in the new National Health Service.[78]

After the war the refugee practitioners gradually entered British medical practice and many of their children followed them into medical careers.[79] The 352 doctors who had obtained the Scottish Triple Qualification had cause to be grateful to the Examination Board for their determination to maintain the existing regulations. In particular they were grateful to John Orr in Edinburgh

Table 7:3 Careers of German Licentiates

	No.	%
General Practice	60	37.3
Internal Medicine	20	12.4
Psychiatry and Psychoanalysis	13	8.1
Surgery	12	7.4
Private Practice	11	6.9
Radiology	6	3.7
M.O.H.	6	3.7
Paediatrics	6	3.7
Obstetrics/Gynaecology	5	3.1
Bacteriology/Pathology	5	3.1
Dermatology	4	2.5
Others	14	8.7
TOTAL	162	100.0

Data obtained from Medical Directories for refugee physicians who obtained the Triple Qualification between 1934-1945.

and Dr. Grant at Glasgow Royal Infirmary who were equally determined that clinical teaching should be made available to the newcomers.

Scottish psychiatrists like Dr. Peter McGowan in Dumfries,Dr. Winifred Rushforth in Edinburgh and Dr. Angus MacNiven in Glasgow had given refugee psychiatry and psychoanalysis the chance to flourish, and in making use of the skills of William Meyer-Gross and Erwin Stengel they served their hospitals well. Michael Balint, who made an outstanding contribution to the understanding of the doctor-patient relationship, was another refugee pyschiatrist who obtained the Triple Qualification in Edinburgh during the war years.

The support for the refugee physicians by the Scottish extra-mural colleges can only be taken to display genuine humanitarian concern, although buttressed by solid financial support that the additional student body provided. While many of the refugees undoubtedly did hope to move on to other countries, it was likely that many would seek to practise in Britain, in competition with local graduates. They could not be compared to the American students whose aim was to return home to the States as quickly as possible, and in fact only a handful of Americans actually remained in Britain. In addition the Scottish colleges felt bound by an undertaking made to the refugees that their requalification regulations would continue to remain in force.

The Scottish universities did not respond in the manner of the extra-mural colleges constrained as they were by their primary concern of providing a medical education for increasing numbers of local students. They showed their concern in other ways, such as in support of the projects of the SPSL and in setting up the Polish School of Medicine. In any case they were certainly aware of the warm reception being offered to the refugee practitioners by the extra-mural colleges and by the various hospitals who were giving the refugee physicians their first opportunity to practise in Britain.

The Scottish colleges had to be sensitive to the views of their members and fellows and could not have consistently conducted a policy far out of line with the wishes of their membership. The senior members of the medical profession in Scotland, who formed the leadership in the Royal colleges and the hospitals, followed the Scottish pattern set in earlier years of enabling outsiders to obtain British qualifications not easily obtainable elsewhere.

For a few years Scotland was home to about 200 refugee practitioners preparing for their final examinations. For the others, who were able to find places elsewhere for their clinical training, it was only the prospect of the Scottish examinations which gave them the chance to find places to study, and often the will to continue.

As we have seen some of the refugees studied in England but took the Scottish qualifications. However the essential feature of the period was that German medical graduates could take the final examinations of the Triple Qualification Board after only one year. This facility remained constant during the years of the refugee influx and contrasted with the more restrictive policy of the English colleges. In an age of intolerance the hand of friendship was gratefully received.

REFERENCES

1. A. J. Sherman, *Island Refuge: Britain and the Refugees from the Third Reich*, (1973) p.20
2. ibid., p.21
3. ibid., p.23
4. Austin Stevens, *The Dispossessed* (1975) p.123
5. Harry Bloch, 'The Berlin Correspondence in the JAMA During the Hitler Regime', *Bulletin of the History of Medicine*, (1973) p.297
6. W. Personal communication
7. *Jewish Echo* 11 Sept. 1936
8. *Jewish Echo* 20 Aug. 1928
9. *Supplement to the British Medical Journal* 16 Sept. 1933, p.165
10. *Minutes of the General Medical Council for 1934* Vol. LXXX1, pp.160-2
11. *Minutes of the General Medical Council for 1933* Vol. LXXX, pp.130-1
12. The attitudes of the popular press to the admission of foreign doctors is considered in: E. Hearst, 'A Brain Gain Rejected', *Weiner Library Bulletin* Vol. X1X (1965) pp.27-8
13. G. H. Brown, *Munk's Roll, Volume 1V, Lives of the Fellows of the Royal College of Physicians of London* (1955) pp.446-9
14. A. M. Cooke, *A History of the Royal College of Physicians of London*, Vol. 3, (Oxford 1972) pp.1069-72
15. W. S. Craig, *History of the Royal College of Physicians of Edinburgh* (Oxford 1971) pp.349-50
16. A. J. Sherman op.cit., p.48
17. Minutes of this meeting are in HO45/15882/666764, Public Records Office
18. ibid.
19. W. S. Craig, op.cit., pp.349-50
20. Francis Watson, *Dawson of Penn* (1950) pp.286-93
21. Minutes of Meeting of the Medical Committee of 18 Sept. 1933 in *Glasgow Royal Infirmary: Minutes of Meetings of Managers and Committee*, pp.172,191
22. F. E. Personal communication
23. F. C. Personal communication
24. Minutes Books of Anderson's College and St. Mungo's College in Glasgow and of the Governing Board of the School of Medicine of the Royal Colleges, Edinburgh.
25. Sir Charles Illingworth, *University Statesman: Sir Hector Hetherington* (Glasgow 1971) p.55
26. SPSL Memorandum 11 July 1933 in SPSL Records (1933-1951) at the Bodleian Library, Oxford.
27. E. Personal communication
28. 'University of Glasgow Regulation of Admission to the Pathology Department of the Glasgow Royal Infirmary: 2 May 1937' in *Minute Book of St. Mungo's College, 1914-1941*
29. Meeting of the Admission Committee of the Medical School of the Royal Colleges, Edinburgh; held in the Dean's office on Saturday 3 June 1933
30. SPSL Records (1933-1951) (Medicine: Individual files) Bodleian Library, Oxford
31. S. L. Personal communication
32. Obituary of Herbert Herxheimer in BMJF, 4 Jan. 1986 '... the most expedient course was the Scottish triple qualification and he approached the pathology with some trepidation. The examiner beamed at him, placed a pot on the table

and said, 'With a name like yours I suppose I dont have to tell you what that is?' Hx. said, 'Gumma', and the rest of the viva was purely social.'
33 H. F. Personal communication
34 SPSL Records (1933-1951) (Medicine: Individual files), Bodleian Library, Oxford.
35 A. J. Sherman op.cit., p.26
36 M. W. Personal communication
37 E. Personal communication
38 Walter Adams, 'The Refugee Scholars of the 1930's, *The Political Quarterly*, Vol. 39, No. 1, pp.7-14
39 Lord Beveridge, *A Defence of Free Learning* (1959)
40 Archives of the Society for the Protection of Science and Learning:Medicine:- Individual files
41 See obituaries in the *BMJ*, eg. L.S. 20 Sept. 1975 ; personal communication, W.S., F.C.
42 E. Hearst op.cit., pp.27-8
43 Editorial, 'As Others See Us', *Lancet* 4 Feb. 1939, pp.274-5
44 *BMJ* 30 May 1938, pp.268-9
45 *BMJ* 9 July 1938, p.79
46 Lord Templewood (Sir Samuel Hoare), *Nine Troubled Years* (1954) p.239
47 Frank Honigsbaum, *The Division in British Medicine* (1979) p.276
48 ibid., p.277
49 A. J. Sherman op.cit., p.108
50 Samson Wright, 'Our Colleagues in Austria', letter, *Lancet* 9 April 1938, p.865
51 SPSL Records (1933-1951), Bodleian Library, Oxford
52 Sir Charles Illingworth op.cit., p.55
53 Sir Charles Illingworth, personal communication
54 Medical Faculty and Senate Minutes, Aberdeen University
55 Samson Wright, 'Our Colleagues in Austria', letter, *Lancet* 9 April 1938, p.865
56 Editorial, 'As Others See Us', *Lancet* 4 Feb. 1939, pp.274-5
57 Kenneth E. Collins, 'Angus MacNiven and the Austrian Psychoanalysts', *Glasgow Medicine* Vol.2 No.5 (1985) pp.18-19
58 Allan C. Tait, *Review of Clinical Services (at Crichton Royal)*, in Dumfries and Galloway Health Board Archives, pp.5-7
59 Aubrey Lewis, 'William Mayer-Gross: An Appreciation' *Psychological Medicine* (1977) Vol. 7, pp.11-18
60 Allan C. Tait op.cit., p.8
61 David Hamilton, *The Healers* (Edinburgh 1982) p.225
62 *Minutes of the General Medical Council for the Year 1941*, Vol. LXXVll (1941) pp.82-3
63 *Minutes of the General Medical Council for the Year 1941*, Vol. LXVlll (1942) pp.4-5, 50-1
64 see Peter and Leni Gillman, *Collar the Lot: How Britain Interned and Expelled its Wartime Refugees* (1980)
65 Lord Templewood op.cit., p.241
66 E. Personal communcation
67 J. A. Personal communication
68 H. E. Personal communication
69 E. Hearst op.cit., pp.27-8
70 Austin Stevens, op.cit., p.130
71 *Lewis Rifkind* (published by the Lewis Rifkind Memorial Book Committee in Conjunction with Glasgow Poale Zion) n.d., p.17

72 E. G. Personal communication
73 see Desider Engel, *Pages of a Surgeon's Diary* (Jerusalem, 1984) pp.241-63
74 see J. Rostowski, *History of the Polish School of Medicine: University of Edinburgh* (University of Edinburgh 1955)
75 Arthur Ruppin, *The Jews in the Modern World* (1934) pp.312-15
76 Letter from British Embassy, Warsaw to Lord Halifax, 1938 FO370/C14496
77 Frank Honigsbaum op.cit., p.313
78 article from *Manchester Guardian*, reprinted in *Association of Jewish Refugees Information* February 1946, p.11
79 Personal communication, on file

Conclusion

The openness and flexibility of Scottish education from the eighteenth century until the middle of the twentieth century benefitted generations of Jews and gave Scottish Jewry the opportunity for substantial involvement in the medical profession. Thus Jewish and Scottish needs neatly coincided. Jews were amongst the first medical graduates in Scotland and included some of the early students in medicine at the University of Edinburgh. Jewish involvement, therefore, follows the development of Scottish medicine. In addition, the history of Jews and medicine in Scotland parallels the course of contemporary Jewish history from the Portuguese Inquisition in the eighteenth century to the Nazi persecutions of the 1930's and 1940's. Both these groups of immigrants to Britain included a number of medical practitioners and the professional element within Anglo-Jewry as a whole increased as the community became more prosperous, established and acculturated.

In the eighteenth and nineteenth centuries Scottish medical education, based in Edinburgh but with increasing competition from Glasgow, was able to accommodate students from a wide variety of religious and national backgrounds. With the Scottish universities usually in a precarious situation there was always a welcome extended to prospective students. Thus Scottish medicine thrived on its continuing international attraction.

I have been able to illustrate the receptive nature of the Scottish universities and medical schools over these two centuries. This gave the chance to a small immigrant group to improve their social status by entering the medical profession. The Jewish doctors did not, however, enter the elites of the medical profession but found careers in the provinces, in army and colonial service and in work within the Jewish community. By the twentieth century, with the rise of State medicine, there were more opportunities for stable medical employment in the growing ranks of the general practitioners. In addition a small number of Scottish Jews managed to become hospital consultants and medical professors.

The transformation of the condition of Jews in Britain after the great wave of immigration which began in the 1880's led to the formation of large groups of Jews in the poorest areas of Britain's industrial cities, engaged in such activities as peddling and sweat-shop trades. I have been able to show that the Jewish parents' dream of their son's entry into the medical profession could indeed become a reality in Scotland. Gorbals Jewry and the children of the tailors, pedlars and cabinetmakers were well represented amongst Glasgow Jewish medical students.

The Scottish universities had a tradition of seeking out promising children and giving them positive help. With parental support, and the financial backing of Carnegie grants, the ladder of opportunity reached the sons of the Jewish immigrants as well as the sons of those Jews who had already achieved a degree of success in Scotland. Scottish Jews created a close-knit community based on mutual aid and self-help against attacks from outside, such as the threat posed by the Christian missionaries. Education and adaptation to Scottish norms was one of the immigrant priorities and for those capable of further advancement this was seen to be best achieved through the medium of medical study.

In the 1930's when the large majority of Jewish students in Scotland were studying medicine, there were alternative study possibilities, especially in teaching and the law. However, the parochial nature of a Scottish law degree as compared to the international character of medicine, taken together with the perceived difficulties of entering the conservative Scottish law firms, meant that medicine had no serious challenger. While teaching was more popular in the 1930's amongst Scots Jews compared to the situation a decade earlier it never achieved the status enjoyed by the medical profession.

The way into the medical profession was led by the sons of the Jewish clergy, which was the community's first professional grouping. The rabbinate in Scotland did not receive the respect accorded to religious leadership in Eastern Europe and was not seen as a suitable career to the aspiring Jewish professional.

This determination to enter medicine was not solely a feature of Scottish Jewry but occurred throughout the contemporary Jewish world where opportunities for higher education were available. The great Jewish thirst for education and a medical training led to the development of quotas in certain American medical schools. Increasing numbers of American Jews, for the American medical students overseas were almost all Jews, found their way to Scotland and other countries. The Scottish group formed an increasing proportion of the American medical students abroad as the 1930's progressed.

By the twentieth century the Scottish medical schools were facing new challenges. The number of Scots entering medicine was increasing although as late as the early 1930's there was still unrestricted access to the Scottish medical schools. Even after the English medical schools stopped admitting American medical students, following the discussions at the GMC, the path to the Scottish universities remained open. The numbers of American students only began to fall as the size of the medical faculties in Glasgow and Edinburgh were stabilised at a level which involved increasing competition for places among local students. In St. Andrews University the Medical Faculty grew as the Americans flocked to classes in St. Andrews and Dundee.

The overseas students found in the extra-mural medical colleges, institutions which continued the Scottish traditions of accommodating foreign students in considerable numbers. The Americans gained from their studies in Scotland. They learned the skills of clinical observation and bed-side diagnosis although Scottish medical science was considered to be less well advanced as compared to American developments. The very success of the Scottish colleges in attracting American students, and their providing the opportunities for refugee practitioners to enter British medicine, may actually have led to their decline. Their burgeoning rolls were accompanied by the expansion of their activities into those teaching hospitals where facilities were being curtailed for the local university students.

The Scottish colleges and the Triple Qualification Board provided the easiest way for the refugee practitioners to enter British medicine. They were prepared to stand up to pressure from their London counterparts who expected them to fall into line with plans to make the obtaining of a British medical licence much harder. Thus it was primarily in Scotland that Jewish medical refugees from Nazi Germany were able to obtain the medical diplomas which would enable them to enter British medicine.

The Scottish universities were unable to provide more than token support for the refugees in the 1930's although such activities as those of the SPSL had their counterparts in Scotland. In addition the later development of a Polish School of Medicine at the University of Edinburgh was an unique development at a dark period of world history. However, the Scottish extramural colleges proved able to cope with the influx of both the Americans and the continental refugees and the flexibility of the facilities they offered proved to be more useful than those which could have been offered by the universities.

The move of British Jews into the professions which had begun substantially in the inter-war years accelerated after the Second World War and the former medical preponderance gradually gave way to a more even spread of Jewish students through the different professional groupings.[1] Occupationally, Anglo-Jewry continued to be divided into two major groupings, namely the professional and the business/management with the former group being often the descendants of the later immigrants who were mostly self-employed or manual workers.[2] The latter group in business and management followed the family mercantile tradition though often enlarging the original businesses and becoming economically more successful. Thus post-war developments were built on the foundations laid a generation or two earlier.

The basis for this successful transformation of Scottish Jewry emerged in the inter-war years when a large professional element was formed in all the Scottish Jewish communities. Medicine was the route out of the ghetto for hundreds of Scottish Jews and their achievements led the way for the greater professionalisation of the community. With the increasing professional element came the successful integration of Scottish Jewry into the society of the host community.

This Jewish penetration of the medical profession over a period of two hundred years through the use of Scottish facilities, has many implications. The successful Jewish professional advancement showed that social mobility could be achieved through the Scottish educational system. The Scottish meritocratic tradition in education, drew in a generation of Jews seeking professional qualifications and sustained their social improvement. In addition the medical schools in Scotland proved to be permeable enough to provide educational opportunities for successive generations of overseas Jews.

The story of the Jews in medicine in Scotland draws together many diverse strands in the Jewish experience. The group social mobility achieved by the

Jews in medicine in Scotland enabled the new medical graduates to make their own way in their future professional life with the possibilities limited only by the difficulties they would encounter in their chosen career.

REFERENCES

1 Harold Pollins, *Economic History of the Jews in England* (1982) pp.234-5
2 Barry A. Kosmin, 'Localism and Pluralism in British Jewry 1900-1980', *TJHSE*, Vol. XXVIII (1984) p.117

Appendices

APPENDIX I. Biographical Index of Jewish medical students and graduates in Scotland before 1880, and Jewish doctors providing affidavits for degrees *in absentia*.

1. EDWIN ADOLPHUS M.D. (Edin.)

A medical student at Edinburgh University from 1834 to 1838, he graduated in 1838 with M.D. from Edinburgh University with a thesis entitled 'On the pathological characters of urine as indicating the presence and extent of disease'.

2. SIR JACOB ADOLPHUS M.D. (c.1775-1845)

A native of Jamaica, he joined the army in 1798 and as a reward for army service in various medical departments he was knighted in 1840. He held the rank of Inspector General of Army Hospitals and Physician General to the Militia Forces on Jamaica. His commission with the rank of Major-General was dated December, 1832. He was a member of the Board of Health on Jamaica. In 1816 he had received the degree of M.D. from Marischal College, Aberdeen with recommendations from local Jamaican physicians and he himself provided an affidavit for another Jamaican colleague for the medical diploma from Marischal College. He was a Member of the Royal College of Surgeons of England in 1817 and was admitted as Fellow in 1840. He died at Cheltenham in Gloucestershire in 1845.
Reference: J. A. P. M. Andrade, *Record of the Jews in Jamaica* (Kingston 1941) pp.148-9

3. CHARLES ASHENHEIM M.D. (Edin.) (1828-1866)

The younger brother of Louis Ashenheim (q.v.) whom he followed in undertaking medical studies at the University of Edinburgh. He had a long and interrupted medical undergraduate career between 1843 and 1852 and was finally awarded his M.D. in 1852 with a thesis on 'delirium tremens', at which time he had already been admitted as Licentiate of the Royal College of Surgeons of Edinburgh. He emigrated to New South Wales practising in the town of Dubbo where he died in 1866.
Reference: A. Levy, *Origins of Scottish Jewry* (1958) pp.14-15. Personal communication, Australian Jewish Historical Society, 1983.

4. LOUIS ASHENHEIM M.D. (St. A) (1816-1858)

The first Scottish born Jewish medical graduate and older brother of Charles Ashenheim (q.v.), he was born in Edinburgh the son of Jacob Ashenheim and Malky Aaron, his father having immigrated from Holland and, being a jeweller to trade, was admitted a burgess in Edinburgh in 1828. He studied at Edinburgh University from 1834 to 1837 but did not graduate there, receiving his M.D. from St. Andrews University, being the first Jew to do so. He was admitted a Licentiate of the Royal College of Surgeons of Edinburgh and practised for a time in London where he first became interested in journalism, being a contributor and then sub-editor of the *Voice of Jacob*. After paying lengthy professional visits to Paris and Berlin he emigrated to Jamaica in 1843. He practised initially in Kingston and later in Falmouth where he encouraged public health measures by lecture and pamphlet and rendered valuable services during a cholera outbreak. In Jamaica he continued with journalistic activities editing the local Jewish journal *Bikkurei Hayam* and he was editor and proprietor of the Jamaican paper *Daily Gleaner*. He was active in the Freemasons in Jamaica serving as Master of the Friendly Lodge of Kingston.

References: A. Levy, *Origins of Scottish Jewry* (1958) pp.14-15. James Picciotto, *Sketches of Anglo-Jewish History*, ed. Israel Finestein, (1956) pp.401,497. *Encyclopaedia Judaica*, (Jerusalem 1972) Vol. 3, col.699. *Jewish Encyclopaedia*, (New York 1925) Vol. 2, p.178.

5. ASHER ASHER M.D. (Glas.) (1837-1889)

He was born in Glasgow, the son of Philip and Hannah Asher, Polish Jewish immigrants to Scotland. He received his education at St. Enoch's School and the High School of Glasgow. After four years of study, he graduated from the University of Glasgow with the degree of M.D., the first Glasgow born Jew to do so. In 1856, the same year as his graduation, he became a licentiate of the Royal College of Surgeons of Edinburgh. He served as parochial medical officer for Wester Cadder until leaving for London in 1862 when he joined Dr. Jacob Canstatt in London as medical officer to the Jewish Board of Guardians. In 1866 he became secretary of the Great Synagogue and in 1870 became secretary of the newly formed United Synagogue. He was a keen Hebrew scholar and wrote extensively on matters of Jewish and medical interest, being a regular correspondent of the medical and Jewish press. He compiled a lengthy monograph on the rite of circumcision and was strongly opposed to superstition. He died of lung cancer in London in 1889 at the age of only 52.

References: D. Kohn-Zedek, *Some Notes and Articles by Asher Asher M.D* bound with a biographical sketch (in Hebrew) (1916). A. Levy, *The Origins of Glasgow Jewry* (Glasgow 1949) pp.58-9. *Jewish Encyclopaedia* Vol. 2, pp.180-1. Kenneth Collins, 'Asher Asher, Doctor of the Poor', *Glasgow Medicine* No.2, Mar/Apr. 1984, p.12

6. DANIEL BARUH M.D.

A member of a prominent Sephardi family in London, Baruh became the first Jewish graduate at King's College, Aberdeen when he graduated M.D. there in 1816 with recommendations from Dr. Sequira and Dr. Joseph Hart Myers.

7. SIMON BELINFANTE M.D. (St. A.) (c.1830-1874)

Born in Holland where the Belinfante family had settled, after some centuries in the Balkans following departure from Portugal in 1526. He pursued a distinguished undergraduate career where he was an anatomy gold medallist. He was one of the few St. Andrews graduates to receive the M.D. with first class honours. He commenced medical practice in Australia in 1862 beginning in North Queensland after arriving as Ship's Surgeon on the 'Bejapore'. He came to New South Wales in about 1864 and practised medicine in Sydney. In 1868 he also qualified as a barrister and practised both professions. Hesettled in Mudgee during the gold rush period. He died in a drowning accident on the Cudgegong River in 1874 and the place is marked there today by the Belinfante Bridge.

References: J. H. Heaton, *Australian Dictionary of Dates*, (Sydney 1879) p.182. *Encyclopaedia Judaica* (Jerusalem 1972) Vol.4, col.436-7. Personal communication, M. Z. Forbes, President-Editor, Australian Jewish Historical Society.

8. MEYER JOSEPH BERNSTEIN M.D., B.Sc. (1855-1915)

After studying in Edinburgh, Bernstein worked first in Liverpool before settling in Manchester. In Manchester he was physician in skin diseases and was a member of the staff of the Jewish Hospital.

Reference: *Jewish Chronicle* 23 April 1915.

9. DAVID BRAVO (c.1780-1822)

David Bravo came from Jamaica and studied at Edinburgh University in 1808-1809. He married Rachel, daughter of Jacob Guttierez of London and was probably a brother of Moses Bravo (q.v.)

Reference: J. A. P. M. Andrade, *Record of the Jews in Jamaica* (Kingston 1941) p.186

10. MOSES BRAVO (1779-1864)

Moses Bravo also came from Jamaica and studied at Edinburgh University in 1800-1801. He returned to practise in Jamaica where he died in 1864. His tombstone in Kingston refers to him as Dr. Moses Bravo.

Reference: J. A. P. M. Andrade, *Record of the Jews in Jamaica* (Kingston 1941) p.231

11. WILLIAM BRODUM M.D.

A German Jew, he came from Mecklenbergh-Strelitz. He was a London quack who began his career as a footman to the mountebank Dr. Bossy, who had a stall at Covent Garden. The success of his medicines enabled him to move from Albion Street in Blackfriars to the West End. By the time of his naturalisation, by Act of Parliament, he declared himself as possessing the Protestant religion and Dr. Joseph Hart Myers refused to accept his annual subscription to the Jewish school in London on this account.

Reference: C.J.S. Thompson, *The Quacks of Old London* (1928) pp.328-9. John Camp, *The Healer's Art* (1978) pp.87-8. Alfred Rubens, 'Portrait of Anglo-Jewry', *TJHSE* (1959) Vol. 19, p.22. Salmond S. Levin, 'Origins of the Jews' Free School', *TJHSE* (1959) Vol.19, p.102. Kenneth Collins, 'Quack Medicines in the Glasgow Advertiser in 1798' *Scottish Medicine* (December 1983) Vol. 3, pp.10-11

12. SAMUEL CARDOZO M.D. (-1885)

A native of London, Cardozo studied at Guy's Hospital. He graduated from Aberdeen University in 1859 and also held the qualifications of member of the Royal College of

Surgeons of England and was Licentiate of the Society of Apothecaries. He settled to practise in Salisbury after working as resident physician to the St. Andrews Castle Asylum in Suffolk.

13. DAVID COHEN M.D.

One of the first Jewish medical graduates at Marischal College, receiving his M.D. diploma there in 1755 with good attestations from Edinburgh and London. Cohen subsequently left Britain, it is believed, to practise in Africa.

14. DOUGLAS COHEN M.D.

A native of Swansea, where there was a small Jewish community from the early eighteenth century, Cohen studied medicine at Edinburgh University, graduating M.D. there in 1828 with a thesis 'on gangrene'. He returned to Swansea where he practised for a short time before moving on to Liverpool. He was still on the medical register with a Liverpool address in 1880. He subsequently retired to Nice.

15. JOSEPH DA CUNHA M.D.

He graduated M.D. from Marischal College, Aberdeen in 1814 and in the same year was admitted as a licentiate of the Royal College of Surgeons in London. He later practised in Oporto.
Reference: William Munk, *Roll of the Royal College of Physicians of London* (1878) Vol. 3, p.119

16. AARON HART DAVID M.D. (Edin.) (1812-1882)

David was born in Montreal, his grandfather Lazarus David having been born in Swansea and came over to Canada at the time of the British conquest, dying in Montreal in 1776. He received his initial medical training in Canada, being indentured to Dr. William Caldwell in 1829. He entered the Medical Faculty of M'Gill University in its first session in the autumn of 1833. He spent the 1834-5 session at Edinburgh University where he received his M.D. in 1835 with a thesis 'on infanticide'. From 1837-9 he was assistant surgeon with the Montreal Rifles, and from 1841-4 he practised in Three Rivers before returning to Montreal. In 1852, he helped to found the Canadian Medical Journal and from 1870 was Dean of the Faculty of Medicine at the University of Bishop College, later absorbed into M'Gill University. He was one of the original members of the Canadian Medical Association and was elected its general secretary in 1869. He was a licentiate of the Royal College of Surgeons of Edinburgh and was an extra-ordinary member of the Royal Medical Society of Edinburgh. In addition to his work as a physician he also attained distinction for his work as a medical politician and as a journalist.
References: B. G. Sack, *History of the Jews in Canada* (Montreal 1945) Vol. 1, p.60.
   Harry C. Ballon, 'Aaron Hart David M.D.' *Can. Med. Assn. J* 86, (1962) pp.115-122

17. MIGUEL CAETANO DE CASTRO M.D. (Edin.)

Born in Rio de Janeiro, Brazil and studied for a time in Coimbra in Portugal before coming to study and graduate in Edinburgh. After practising for a time in Devonshire he returned to Portugal.
Reference: William Munk, *Roll of the Royal College of Physicians of London* (1878) Vol. 3, p.135

18. JOAO PEREIRA DE CASTRO M.D. (Edin.)

There were members of the Spanish and Portuguese Jews' Congregation in London bearing this surname during the latter half of the eighteenth century.
Reference: Richard Barnett, 'Dr. Jacob de Castro Sarmento and Sephardim in Medical Practice in 18th Century London', *TJHSE*, (1982) Vol.27, p.110

19. PHILIP DE LA COUR (1710-1780)

He was born in London but took his medical degree at Leiden in Holland and he became a licentiate of the Royal College of Physicians of London in 1751. He was the uncle of Dr. Sequira with whom he initially practised in London before moving to Bath, where he died in 1780. He provided an affidavit for a candidate for the degree of M.D. at Marischal College, Aberdeen and was quoted by William Brodum in one of his advertisements in the 'Glasgow Advertiser' of 1798 as a celebrated physician who used Dr. Brodum's Nervous Cordial. He was originally known as Abraham Gomes Ergas, being of Portuguese origins.
Reference: *Jewish Encyclopaedia*, (New York 1925) Vol.11, p.200

20. HANANEL DE LEON M.D. (Edin.)

A native of Jamaica, he came to Edinburgh where he studied medicine from 1816 to 1818, graduating M.D. there in 1818 with a thesis 'on hydrocephalus'. In 1821 he became a licentiate of the Royal College of Physicians of London.
Reference: William Munk, *Roll of the Royal College of Physicians of London* (1978) Vol. 3, p.244

21. SOLOMON DE LEON M.D.

A native of the Caribbean island of St. Kitts, he came to Edinburgh to study for two sessions beginning in 1786. He completed his studies in Holland, graduating M.D. from Leiden with a thesis 'on inflammation'. He became a licentiate of the Royal College of Physicians of London in 1791, and subsequently served as honorary physician to the Hebra (Congregation of Spanish and Portuguese Jews in London), consulting his friends Dr. Sequira and Dr. Myers when needed.
References: R. W. Innes-Smith, *English Speaking Students at the University of Leyden*, (Edinburgh 1932) p.65. Richard Barnett, 'Dr. Jacob de Castro Sarmento and Sephardim in Medical Practice in 18th Century London', *TJHSE* (1982) Vol. 27, p.112. William Munk, *Roll of the Royal College of Physicians of London* (1878) Vol. 2, p.418

22. MAURICE DAVIS M.D. (St. A.) (1821-1898)

He was educated at King's College, London, where he had a distinguished undergraduate career, gaining first prize in clinical medicine and surgery. In 1852 he qualified with L.S.A. and M.R.C.S. (England) and in the same year graduated M.D. from St. Andrews University. He played an active part in Jewish communal activities as well as in medical matters and served as a member of the Jewish Board of Guardians, the Anglo-Jewish Association and was honorary Medical Officer of the Jewish Convalescent Home. He served on the metropolitan branch of the British Medical Association, produced some literary work and was active in charitable endeavours.
References: *Jewish Encyclopaedia* (New York 1925) Vol. 4, p.474. *Jewish Chronicle*, obituary on 30th September 1898.

23. LEONARD EMANUEL M.D. (St. A.) (1835-1864)

He pursued his medical studies at University College, London where he won many prizes. In addition to his M.D. from St. Andrews University he held M.R.C.S. (England), L.R.C.P. (London) and L.S.A. He was a member of the Visitation Committee of the Jewish Board of Guardians in London. He accepted a commission in the Indian Medical Service but died at the young age of 29 years from a rapidly fatal form of spinal paralysis, which was written up in the Lancet (1864, Vol.i, p.599).
References: *Annual Report of the Jewish Board of Guardians* (1864). D. G. Crawford, *Roll of the Indian Medical Service 1615-1930* (1930) p.166

24. HENRY FRAENKEL M.D. (Edin.)

Of the family of one of the first Jews to settle in Cape Town, Siegfried Fraenkel, a German Jew who settled at the Cape in 1808 and was active as a surgeon and was among the founders of the Cape Town Synagogue and the South African College. He returned from his years of study in Edinburgh to practise in South Africa.
Reference: Louis Herrman, *History of the Jews in South Africa* (Cape Town 1935) pp.107-15

25. DANIEL GARCIA M.D.

Practised in London after receiving his diploma from King's College, Aberdeen.

26. REUBEN GROSS M.D (Glas.)

Originally from Liverpool, he came to study in Glasgow and graduated there in 1862. In the same year he became a licentiate of the Royal College of Surgeons of Edinburgh. He initially returned to practise in Liverpool but eventually settled in California.

27. JOEL HART L.R.C.S. (England) (1784-1842)

Born in Philadelphia and studied medicine in London before coming to Edinburgh in 1804. He was a member of the Royal Medical Society of Edinburgh. He returned to the United States after being a licentiate of the Royal College of Surgeons of England and was one of the charter memebers of the Medical Society for the County of New York.Additionally, he was an active Mason in New York. He returned to Scotland in

1817, having been appointed United States Consul in Leith, near Edinburgh, by President Madison, a post he held until 1832. Following his final return to America he practised in New York until his death there in 1842.
References: *Jewish Encyclopaedia* (New York 1925) Vol. 6, p.240. *Encyclopaedia Judaica* (Jerusalem 1972) Vol. 7 col.1357

28. JOSEPH GUTTERES HENRIQUES M.R.C.S. (England) (1796-1885)

He was born into a prominent Jewish family on Jamaica, being born in Kingston in 1796. He came to London, commencing his medical studies at St. Thomas's Hospital, going on to Edinburgh University where he was enrolled as a medical student for the 1818-19 session. After becoming a licentiate of the Royal College of Surgeons of England, he returned to Jamaica where he practised as an ophthalmologist. He returned to London to continue his work in eye disease in 1825, marrying there Eliza Bravo, whose family also hailed from Jamaica. He began to practise in London, but never managed to become Consultant Physician at the Ophthalmic Hospital in Finsbury, due it was thought, to anti-Jewish prejudice. He retired from medical practice to devote himself to communal activities and was acting as President of the Board of Deputies of British Jews during the absence from Britain of Sir Moses Montefiore, who was then conducting diplomatic negotiations related to the Damascus 'Blood Libel' of 1840.
Reference: *Jewish Chronicle*, obituary on 11th September 1885.

29. MOSES NUNES HENRIQUES

The first of many Jamaican Jews to study in Scotland, he matriculated as a medical student at Edinburgh University for the session 1789-90. He returned to Jamaica to practise and it was recorded that he was still practising as a physician and surgeon in 1823.
Reference: J. A. P. M. Andrade, *Record of the Jews in Jamaica* (Kingston 1941) p.175

30. SOLOMON IFFLA L.F.P.S. (Glas.) (1816-1886)

Iffla claimed descent from a French Catholic family which traced its origin back to the early Saxon Kings. He was the younger brother of Daniel Osiris Iffla, the famous French benefactor and heir to the Marquis d'If. Daniel Iffla embraced Judaism and was founder of the Sephardi Synagogue in the Rue Buffault in Paris, and it seems likely that Solomon Iffla was also a convert to Judaism. Iffla was born in Bordeaux in 1816 and with Iffla family involvement in the Revolution in 1830, he was sent with his brothers to Scotland, Charles X and his entourage setting up an exiled French Court for a time at Holyrood in Edinburgh. He subsequently emigrated to Jamaica but completed his medical training in Glasgow where he became a licentiate of the Faculty of Physicians and Surgeons after examination in 1844. He settled in Australia in 1851 and married Rachel, daughter of David Israel Pereira of Amsterdam in 1855. He was one of the first Jewish physicians in Melbourne having arrived there from Adelaide in 1853. He served as Mayor of Emerald Hill and as District Coroner and was actively involved in Jewish communal matters in Melbourne, both with the synagogue and Jewish education.

References: *Journal of the Australian Jewish Historical Society* Vol.3,1. L. M. Goldman, *Jews in Victoria in the 19th Century* (Melbourne 1954). Copy of letter (unpublished) on the Iffla family from Dr. Richard Barnett to Dr. A. P. Joseph (English respondent of the Australian Jewish Historical Society) with family documents, on file.

31. JOSEPH MARCUS JOSEPH M.D., C.M., Ll.D. (Glas.) (1826-1886)

A native of India, Joseph came to Glasgow after his medical training at St. George's gaining the degrees of Doctor of Medicine and Master of Surgery from the University of Glasgow in 1852. At the end of his training in London he had become a Member of the Royal College of Surgeons of England and in 1857 became only the second Jewish Fellow of the Royal College of Physicians of Edinburgh. He entered the Indian Medical Service and attained the rank of Deputy Surgeon-General in the Bengal Army. In 1866 he received the honorary degree of Ll.D. from the University of Glasgow. He retired from army service in 1885 and died the following year.

Reference: D. G. Crawford, *Roll of the Indian Medical Service 1615-1930* (1930) p.342

32. LAURENCE ALFRED JOSEPH M.D. (Glas.) (c1810-1840)

Later known as Dr. Joseph Laurence, he was the first Jewish medical undergraduate at the University of Glasgow, where he studied from 1829 to 1831 getting permission to be examined early for the degree of M.D. as his regiment, the 4th Dragoon Guards, were leaving for Ireland. He served in the army as assistant surgeon, retiring on half pay in 1838 and died in 1840.

References: List of Commissioned Medical Officers in the British Army Arthur P. Arnold, 'Anglo-Jewish Wills and Letters of Administration' in *Anglo-Jewish Notabilities* (1949) pp.173,175

33. BENJAMIN LARA M.D. (1769-1847)

He was a member of a prominent Sephardi medical family, his father, who was also named Benjamin Lara, having been appointed doctor to the Hebra in 1770. He was the author of 'A Dictionary of Surgery, or the Young Surgeon's Pocket Assistant'. He was a member of the Corporation of Surgeons of London, surgeon to the Royal Cumberland Freemason's School and surgeon to the Portuguese Hospital. He received the degree of M.D. from Marischal College, Aberdeen in 1802 and became the first Jewish Fellow of the Royal College of Physicians of Edinburgh in 1814. He was appointed a Naval Surgeon on the 26th of March and had an extensive practice in Southsea for many years until his death in 1847.

Reference: Richard Barnett, 'Dr. Jacob de Castro Sarmento and Sephardim in Medical Practice in 18th Century London', *TJHSE* (1982) Vol. 27, p.111

34. BENJAMIN LARA

The son of Benjamin Lara M.D. (q.v.) and the third generation in the family of Lara medical men, he came from Portsmouth to study in Edinburgh for several sessions between 1839 and 1848 but does not appear to have completed his studies and was not in practice when the Medical Register began.

APPENDICES

35. LUIS LEO (-1812)

Leo was a physician practising in Houndsditch in London and was a connection of the Goldsmid family who brought him to London and patronised him on condition that he changed his name. He was a member of a Freemason's Lodge. He was responsible for providing the affidavit for William Brodum's successful application for the degree of M.D. from Marischal College and probably also induced Dr. Saunders to endorse it. His family were traditionally associated with manufacturing quill pens and cigar and sweet merchants. His son Henry married Mary Myers, a native of Boston, at Boston, Lincolnshire in 1822.

References: Cecil Roth, *Rise of Provincial Jewry* (1950) p.33. Kenneth Collins, 'The Jewish Quacks of Old Aberdeen' *Scottish Medicine* (November 1983) Vol. 3, pp.16-18

36. SAMUEL LEVENSTON M.D. (Glas.) (1823-1914)

He was a member of a family noted for medical botany and musical talent in Glasgow and Dublin from the middle of the 19th century. He may have begun practising as a medical botanist even before completing his medical studies at the University of Glasgow where he graduated M.D. in 1859. He spent his medical career in Glasgow and was an active member of the Glasgow Hebrew Congregation serving as trustee when the synagogue in George Street was built in 1858 and again in 1878 when the imposing synagogue at Garnethill was erected.

References: A. Levy, *Origins of Glasgow Jewry* (Glasgow 1949) pp.38,46. Kenneth Collins, 'Early Doctors and Medical Botanists', *Jewish Echo*, 13 Sept. 1985.

37. MICHAEL LEVY

Levy, a matriculated medical student at Edinburgh University in the 1851-2 session, was probably the brother-in-law of Charles Ashenheim (q.v.) and in trade in Edinburgh.

38. GUMPERTZ LEWISOHN M.D. (-1797)

He was also known as George (Mordecai Gumpel) Schnaber and was born in Berlin, where he was regarded as a prodigy in Talmudic study. He took up medical studies and came to London to study under John Hunter. While in England he published 'An Essay on the Blood' in 1776 followed by 'Epidemical Sore Throat' in 1778 and the Hebrew work 'Maamar ha-Torah ve-Hokhmah' in 1779. The Hebrew work caused much controversy and he was regarded with suspicion as a religious innovator. He received the degree of M.D. from Marischal College, Aberdeen in 1775, the same year as his polemical work, directed at the leadership of the Great Synagogue in London, was published. This work, *Tokhaha Gedolah* (The Great Reproof) led to a breakdown in relations within the synagogue and soon after he left for Sweden where he was Court Physician and Professor of Medicine in Upsala with the patronage of King Gustavus 111. He subsequently returned to Germany from Sweden settling in Hamburg where he continued to write extensively on medical matters. He died in Hamburg in 1797 and was buried in the Jewish Cemetery there.

References: Jewish Encyclopaedia (New York 1925) Vol. V111, p.46. Cecil Roth, *The History of the Great Synagogue* (1950) p.152-3

39. HEYMAN LION (c.1760-c.1823)

He was one of the earliest Jewish residents in Edinburgh where he practised as a dentist and chiropodist. He enrolled and studied at Edinburgh University between 1790 and 1795 but was refused a medical qualification by both Edinburgh University and King's College, Aberdeen because of the nature of his medical practice. He is the author of a 438 page book on chiropody, a copy of which is in the Edinburgh University Library.

References: Kenneth Collins, 'The Jewish Quacks of Old Aberdeen' *Scottish Medicine* (November 1983) Vol.3, pp.16-18. A. Levy, *The Origins of Scottish Jewry* (1958) pp.11-12

40. BENJAMIN LYON M.D. (-1797)

Received his M.D. degree from Marischal College, Aberdeen in 1783 and in the same year obtained the qualification of licentiate of the Society of Apothecaries (London). Marischal College believed him to be Jewish but appear to have confused him with Dr. Luis Leo who provided the affidavit for William Brodum.

41. ABRAHAM RAPHAEL MENDES DA COSTA

He must be presumed to be the first Jewish undergraduate at a British University, although no further details of his life or professional activities are available. The Mendes da Costa family were a large and prominent Sephardi family in England at this period with interests in business, science and the arts.

Reference: *Encyclopaedia Judaica* (Jerusalem 1972) Vol. 5, col.985-6

42. HANANEL MENDES DA COSTA (c.1797-1818)

From London, he came to Edinburgh where he studied medicine, being an enrolled student at the University from 1815 to 1818. He was active in student activities while in Edinburgh and served as Senior President of the Royal Medical Society presenting a medical dissertation to fellow members of the Society. However, shortly after returning to London to take up medical practice, he died having already shown much promise in his chosen career.

References: James Gray, *History of the Royal Medical Society 1737-1937* (Edinburgh 1952) p.318. Obituary, *Gentleman's Magazine and Historical Chronicle*, (1818) Vol. LXXXV111,i, p.468

43. JOHN MEYER (1749-1825)

One of the most prolific supplier of affidavits for candidates for M.D. degrees at the two colleges in Aberdeen: 7 at King's College including Daniel Garcia (q.v.) and 2 at Marischal College. He was born in Austria but received his medical training at the University of Strasbourg, returning to practice in Vienna. He travelled widely to extend his medical knowledge, visiting London, Paris and other European centres. He settled in London in 1784 becoming a licentiate of the Royal College of Physicians in that year. He was widely respected, both as a physician and as a classical scholar. He died in Brighton soon after retiring there in 1825.

Reference: Obituary, *Gentleman's Magazine and Historical Chornicle*, (1825) Vol. XLV, pp.372-3

44. JUDAH ISRAEL MONTEFIORE M.D. (d.1827)

A first cousin of Sir Moses Montefiore, he was born in Gibraltar, coming to London where he became a surgeon. He served as Surgeon of the Militia on Jamaica in 1809. Returning to London, he had a dispensary in Leman Street. He served as physician to the Sephardi Synagogue in London at an initial salary of £30 per annum. He obtained the M.D. from King's College, Aberdeen in 1824 with attestations by Dr. Frampton and Dr. John Meyer. He emigrated to Jamaica in 1825 and died there in 1827. His son achieved high office in the service of the East India Company.

References: 'Lucien Wolf in Conversation with Joseph Barrow Montefiore', *Essays in Jewish History* (1934) p.32. A. M. Hyamson, *The Sephardim of England* (1951) p.368. J. A. P. M. Andrade, *A Record of the Jews on Jamaica* (Kingston 1941) p.176

45. JOSEPH HART MYERS M.D. (Edin.) (1758-1823)

He was born in New York in 1758 the son of Naphtali Hart Myers who had been Warden of the Great Synagogue in London. He began his education in New York but came to London to continue his studies and to commence his medical education at the lectures of William Hunter and George Fordyce. He came to Edinburgh in 1775 and studied in the Medical Faculty in the University of Edinburgh for four sessions, graduating M.D. there in 1779, after a private and public examination and a defence of his thesis 'on diabetes'. He was the first Jewish graduate at Edinburgh University and was the first Jew to graduate in a British university after completing a regular course of undergraduate studies. After graduation he paid extended professional visits to Leiden, Paris, Vienna and Berlin returning to London where he settled to practise. He was a colleague of Dr. Lettsom on the dispensary at Aldersgate Street and despite being an Ashkenazi with close family links with the Great Synagogue, he was elected to serve as physician to the Hebra (Sephardi Congregation in London). He was a member of the Medical Society of London, serving as librarian and is included in Samuel Medley's painting of members of the society in 1800. He served as President of the London Talmud Torah and was responsible for many improvements in the level of provision of Jewish elementary education in London in the institution which developed into the Jews' Free School. He became a licentiate of the Royal College of Physicians in 1787. His latter years were characterised by his affliction with gout which eventually prevented his carrying out his professional duties. He died in London in 1823.

References: T. Hunt (Editor), *The Medical Society of London 1773-1973* (1972) pp.22-9. A. Levy, *The Origins of Scottish Jewry* (1958) pp. 10-11. William Munk, *Roll of the Royal College of Physicians of London* (1878) Vol. 2, p.376

46. LEVI MYERS M.D. (Glas.) (c.1765-1827)

Levi Myers came from South Carolina to study medicine in Edinburgh and matriculated there for three sessions from 1786 to 1788. After two years of study in Edinburgh he received the degree of M.D. from the University of Glasgow after examination there, being the first Jew to graduate from the University of Glasgow, in September 1787. He returned to Edinburgh for his last year of studies, on completion of which he returned to South Carolina, practising in Charlestown and Georgetown. He was elected to the State Legislature and from 1799 was Apothecary-General for South Carolina, a post he held until his death. He was noted in 1801 as being a prominent physician in Georgetown and was a member of the South Carolina Medical Society. He, his wife and four children all died at sea on 22nd September 1827.

References: Charles Reznikoff, *The Jews of Charlestown* (Philadelphia 1950) p.281. Bernard Elzas, *The Jews of South Carolina* (Philadelphia 1905) pp.128,243. Solomon R. Kagan, *Jewish Contributions to Medicine in America* (Boston 1939) pp.3,485,555. Kenneth Collins, 'The Tale of Doctor Levi Myers', *Glasgow Medicine* May/June 1985 Vol. 2, No. 3, pp.12-13

47. EMANUEL DE ASHER PACIFICO M.D.

A relative of Don Pacifico, on whose behalf Lord Palmerston sent British gunboats to Greece, Emanuel Pacifico was a popular doctor in London with a practice in Bury Street. He obtained the M.D. at King's College, Aberdeen in 1817 with recommendations from Dr. Joseph Hart Myers as well as from Drs. Sutherland and Babington. He served as physician to the Hebra and endowed the almshouses that were known by his name.

References: A. M. Hyamson, *The Sephardim of England* (1951) p.268 'Lucien Wolf in conversation with Joseph Barrow Montefiore', *Essays in Jewish History* (1934) p.32

48. JACOB DE CASTRO SARMENTO M.D. (1691-1762)

He was born as Henrique de Castro in Braganca in northern Portugal to New Christian parents who had been arrested by the Inquisition in 1708. He graduated M.A. from the University of Evora and graduated M.D. from the University of Coimbra in 1717 after 6 years of study. After working in southern Portugal and subsequently in Lisbon, where he probably participated in secret Jewish activity, he left Portugal in 1720. Some believe that he left the country in flight from the Inquisition, settling in London. In 1725 he obtained a licence to practise becoming a licentiate of the Royal College of Physicians. He wrote many medical treatises and, especially in his early years in London, published many works defending his Jewish beliefs. He was appointed doctor of the Hebra in 1724 but was dismissed within a year for 'having written on Passover and ridden in a coach on the 8th day of Tabernacles'. He became a Fellow of the Royal Society in 1730. He was a lifelong and implacable enemy of Dr. Meyer Schomberg who accused him of obtaining his freedom from the Inquisition by betraying others. In 1735 he published his major work on materia medica and at the same period also wrote poetry and a work on the tides. In 1738 he took Dr. Meyer Schomberg to the Disciplinary Committee of the Royal College of Physicians because Schomberg had accused him of dangerous medical treatment. Sarmento was successful and Schomberg was fined £4.

In 1739 Sarmento became the first Jew to receive a university degree in Britain when he was awarded the M.D. by Marischal College, Aberdeen with affidavits from Sir Hans Sloane, then President of the Royal Society, Dr. Cromwell Mortimer and Dr. Alexander Stewart. In 1758 he withdrew from the Synagogue in Bevis Marks and in the following year he married his Christian mistress. His writing included many works on fevers and he introduced into England a medicine called 'Agoas de Inglaterra' which was very successful financially and which was based on the drug quinine.

Within the Jewish community his most lasting monument was the Bet Holim, the hospital of the Hebra, which from the outset was the first in England to include beds for maternity cases. He was, therefore, a scholar of great ability, a skilful physician and writer although he was always living in the midst of great controversy.

References: *Encyclopaedia Judaica*, (Jerusalem 1972) Vol. 5, col.246-7. Harry Friedenwald, *Jews and Medicine* (Baltimore 1944) Vol. 2, pp.457-9. Richard Barnett, 'Dr. Jacob de Castro Sarmento and Sephardim in 18th century practice in London', *TJHSE* (1982) Vol. XXV11, pp.84-103

49. MEYER LOEW SCHOMBERG (1690-1761)

Born in Fetzburg in Germany he was one of the first Jews to be accepted at a German university, receiving the degree of M.D. from the University of Geissen in 1710. He settled in London, becoming a licentiate of the Royal College of Physicians in 1722 and a Fellow of the Royal Society in 1726. He was one of the foremost physicians of his day building up a fashionable clientele as well as acting as physician to the Great Synagogue. He held somewhat unorthodox religious views and he was the author of a polemical work criticising the leaders of the Jewish community for religious hypocrisy. He continued a personal feud with Dr. Jacob de Castro Sarmento (q.v.). He gradually withdrew from the Jewish community in London in the 1740's. Schomberg acted as sponsor for several candidates for the degree of M.D. at Marischal College, Aberdeen, including his son Ralph who received his degree in 1745. His descendants included distinguished naval officers, e.g. Admiral Sir Alexander Wilmot Schomberg (1774-1850). One writer described him as quarrelsome, avaricious, ungenerous, insincere and entirely self-centred and self-satisfied.

References: *Encyclopaedia Judaica* (Jerusalem 1972) Vol. 14, col.992-4. Edgar R. Samuel, 'Anglo-Jewish Notaries and Scriveners', *TJHSE* (1953) Vol. XV11, p.118. Edgar R. Samuel, 'Dr. Meyer Schomberg's Attack on the Jews of London', *TJHSE* (1964) Vol.XX, pp.83-100. Meyer Schomberg, 'Emunat Omen', (trans. Harold Levy), *TJHSE* (1964) Vol. XX, pp.101-11

50. RALPH SCHOMBERG M.D. (1714-1792)

The son of Meyer Schomberg (q.v) and twin brother of Isaac Schomberg who maintained a long running dispute with the Royal College of Physicians. Ralph Schomberg studied medicine at the University of Rotterdam in Holland and sent for his M.D. at Marischal College, Aberdeen from there. The records of Marischal College show that the dues for the diploma were not paid until Schomberg himself cleared the debt when practising in Yarmouth in 1752. From 1761 he practised in Bath and later worked in Pangbourne and Reading. He was a voluminous writer and was said to have been 'a scribbler without genius or veracity'. He plagiarised extensively and was found guilty of disreputable money transactions and literary thefts. He gradually abandoned Jewish life, his eldest son Isaac being baptised as a child. He had been educated at Merchant Taylor's School, the only public school at the time to accept Jewish boys, having also Hebrew on the curriculum. Schomberg died in 1792 and was buried at St. Mary's in the East.

References: *Encyclopaedia Judaica* (Jerusalem 1972) Vol. 14, col.994. Edgar R. Samuel, 'Anglo-Jewish Notaries and Scriveners', *TJHSE* (1953) Vol. XV11, pp.118-19

51. ISAAC HENRIQUE SEQUIRA (1738-1816)

Born in Lisbon, he studied in Bordeaux and then at the University of Leiden where he took his degree in 1758. He settled in London and became a licentiate of the Royal College of Physicians in 1771. He practised with Dr. Philip de la Cour (q.v.), his uncle, who soon after removed to Bath. He held a great reputation in the Jewish community in London and held honorary appointments to the Portuguese Embassy and the Prince Regent of Portugal. At the time of his death he was the oldest College licentiate. He supplied the affidavit for Daniel Baruh's M.D. at King's College, Aberdeen. There is a brief description of him in Israel Zangwill's *Children of the Ghetto*, (1892) as pompous in white stockings.

References: Jewish Encyclopaedia (New York 1925) Vol. X1, p.200. William Munk, *Roll of the Royal College of Physicians of London* (1878) Vol. 2, p.291. 'Lucien Wolf in conversation with Joseph Barrow Montefiore', *Essays in Jewish History* (1934) p.32

52. ABRAHAM SOLOMON M.D. (Edin.) (1790-1827)

The son of the great Liverpool quack Samuel Solomon (q.v.).Abraham came to Edinburgh to study medicine in 1804 while still only 14 years old. He completed his studies in 1810 graduating M.D. from the University of Edinburgh with a thesis 'de cerebri tumoribus'. He married Helen Tyrie and they had 9 children. With his inherited fortune he did not require to practice medicine.

Reference: A. E. Franklin, *Records of the Franklin Family* (1935) pp.117-8

53. SAMUEL SOLOMON M.D. (1745-1819)

He was born in Cork in Ireland the younger son of the Cork shochet, Abraham Solomon. In about 1768 he moved to Dublin where he opened a depot for the sale of his remedies and by 1790 he had moved to Liverpool where he started to popularise his medicine 'The Cordial Balm of Gilead'. He obtained the M.D. from Marischal College, Aberdeen with affidavits from two Liverpool doctors, Dr. Fisher and Dr. Moore. Marischal College had some suspicion afterwards that the affidavits had been obtained by forgery. The diploma and degree were displayed prominently in his publications and in the advertisements promoting his wares. In one advertisement in the *Glasgow Advertiser* he describes himself as a Member of the College of Physicians of Aberdeen (sic). His activities brought him a fortune with world wide sales and he was able to live in style with a mansion (Gilead House) in the Kensington district of Liverpool and many streets in the area were named in his honour (Solomon St., Balm St., Gilead St.). He appears to have had little contact with the Liverpool Jewish community and made burial arrangements with the Jewish community in Manchester. However, he subsequently severed all connections with Judaism 'except in distant sympathy'.

References: Jewish Encyclopaedia (1925) Vol. X1, p.457. Louis Hyman, *The Jews of Ireland* (1972) pp.76-7. Bill Williams, *The Making of Manchester Jewry* (Manchester 1976) pp.14-16. B. L. Benas, *Records of Jews in Liverpool* (Liverpool 1900) pp.13-16. A. E. Franklin, *Records of the Franklin Family* (1935) p.117-8. C. J. S. Thomson, *The Quacks of Old London* (1928) pp.329-332. Kenneth Collins, 'The Jewish Quacks of Old Aberdeen', *Scottish Medicine* (November 1983) Vol. 3, pp.16-18

APPENDICES 177

54. MORITZ STERN M.R.C.S., L.R.C.P. (London) (1833-1890)

He was born in Kingston, Jamaica and came to Edinburgh to study medicine, being a matriculated medical student at the University there from 1854 to 1859. After leaving Edinburgh he took his qualifications in London and returned to Jamaica to practise in 1860. He was surgeon to the Militia on Jamaica in 1865 and became President of the Jamaican branch of the British Medical Association in 1884. He removed to Panama City where he died after practising there for several years.
Reference: J. A. P. M. Andrade, Record of the Jews in Jamaica (Kingston 1941) p.175

55. GEORGE CHARLES WALLACH M.D. (Edin.) (1815-1899)

The son of the distinguished physician and botanist Nathaniel Wallich (q.v.) he was born in India and came to Edinburgh, studying medicine at the University of Edinburgh and graduating there, after 4 years of study, in 1836 with a thesis 'on pneumonia'. He became a licentiate of the Royal College of Surgeons of Edinburgh in 1837 and in the following year he entered the Indian Medical Service. He received medals for his services in the Sutlej and Punjab campaigns of 1842 and 1847 and was field-surgeon during the Sonthal rebellion of 1855-6. He researched extensively over many years in the field of marine biology publishing works on deep sea animals. He received the gold medal of the Linnean Society for his work.
Reference: Dictionary of National Biography (Oxford 1917) Vol. 20, p.593

56. NATHANIEL WALLICH M.D. (1786-1854)

He was born in Copenhagen and was originally known as Nathan Woolff. He studied in Copenhagen and qualified in 1806 as a licentiate of the Royal Academy of Surgeons of Copenhagen. After completing his studies he became surgeon at the Danish settlement of Serampore in India. When the settlement fell into British hands in 1813 Wallich entered into medical service with the British. During this time he travelled extensively, cultivating his great interest in the flora of India. He was appointed superintendent of the Calcutta botanical gardens in 1815 and in 1819 received the degree of M.D. from Marischal College in Aberdeen. He became a Fellow of the Royal Society in 1829. He continued to travel widely throughout the Indian sub-continent exploring Assam, Hindustan and Burma and he catalogued many thousands of species of Indian flora. He was on the original staff of Calcutta Medical College and became Professor of Botany there in 1835. He wrote widely with works printed in botanical and medical journals as well as in the Edinburgh Philosophical Journal. He returned to England in 1847 and resigned his post in 1850 maintaining an active interest in the Linnean Society. An obelisk was erected to his memory in the Calcutta botanical gardens by the East India Company. The Wallich family is a noted Jewish medical family, having produced many distinguished physicians since the 14th century, among them Moshe Wallich, founder of the Shaare Tzedek hospital in Jerusalem, and Otto Wallich, the Nobel Prizewinner. His son, George Charles Wallich, was a graduate of the University of Edinburgh.
References: Dictionary of National Biography (Oxford 1917) Vol. 20, pp.592-3. Encyclopaedia Judaica (Jerusalem 1972) Vol.15 col.1351, Vol.16 col.256-7. D. G. Crawford, History of the Indian Medical Service (1934) Vol. 1, pp.143-4, 147,211,439

57. HART WESSELS (d.1765)

He was one of the first Ashkenazi doctors in Britain, possibly having originated in Hamburg. In 1758 he was formally appointed to attend the poor of the congregation of the Great Synagogue in London at an initial salary of £10 per annum. He tried, unsuccessfully in 1745 and again the following year, to become doctor to the Hebra after a brief appointment as locum tenens for four months. He obviously bore the Hebra no grudge leaving them £200 in his will. He was held in high regard as a physician in Aberdeen, according to the Marischal College records, and was responsible for providing 5 affidavits for doctors seeking the degree of M.D. at Marischal College. However, after his recommendation of Dr. Walker, a purveyor of patent medicine, he was told that his recommendations would not be accepted in Aberdeen any longer. He replied that he had previously given preference to Marischal College but would send them no more applications. Marischal College Fasti record that he was 'a little doubtful with respect to nostrums but in a great deal of credit as a physician in London'.

References: Richard Barnett, 'Dr. Jacob de Castro Sarmento and Sephardim in Medical Practice in 18th Century London', TJHSE (1982) Vol. 27, pp.111,113. Cecil Roth, *The History of the Great Synagogue* (1950) p.85.

58. ALEXANDER ZEIGLER M.D. (St. A.)

Member of a family of jewellers in Edinburgh early in the 19th century. It is thought that the family were of Jewish origin. He became a licentiate of the Royal College of Surgeons in Edinburgh in 1816 and gained the M.D. at St. Andrews University in 1845. He became a Fellow of the Royal College of Physicians of Edinburgh in 1853. He was Consultant Surgeon of the Maternity Hospital in Edinburgh having been Surgeon General of the Lying In Hospital and Dispensary. His son, William, who was also an obstetrician, gained the M.D. of Edinburgh University in 1849, by which time he had become a member of the Free Church.

References: Abel Phillips, *A History of the Origins of the First Jewish Community in Scotland—Edinburgh 1816* (Edinburgh 1979) p.43. Medical Directories Obituary, *Edinburgh Medical Journal* (Edinburgh 1891) Vol. XXXV11, pp.973-6.

APPENDIX II. Questionnaire sent to American Jewish graduates of Scottish medical schools

QUESTIONNAIRE

Name:

Present medical post:
(or last post before retiral)

1. Reasons for not studying medicine in America:

2. How information about Scottish medical school was obtained:

3. Acceptance at medical school:
Place of study ....

4. Memories of medical studies in Scotland:

5. Contacts with local Jewish community:

6. Problems with registering to practise in US:

7. Ease of finding employment with Scottish qualifications:

8. Comments:

APPENDIX III.   Questionnaire sent to German graduates holding the Scottish Triple Qualification

QUESTIONNAIRE

Name:

Present medical post:
(or last post before retiral)

1. Reasons for leaving Europe:

2. Reception in Britain:

3. Acceptance at medical school:
Place of study ....

4. Memories of medical studies in Britain:

5. Problems with Conjoint Board and Requalification:

6. Ease in finding employment:

7. War-time Medical Service:

8. Comments:

Glossary

Glossary of Jewish Terms

Beth Din: religious court usually concerned with kashrut and matters of personal status

Beth Hamedrash: prayer or study house, usually attached to a synagogue

Cheder (plural:chadarim): elementary class in Hebrew and Jewish religious studies

Dayan: Rabbi acting as a religious judge in the Beth Din

Chevra Kadisha: literally, holy fellowship. Name of a Glasgow synagogue but often applied to a Hebrew burial society

Chasidism: pietistic movement which developed in Judaism in the eighteenth and nineteenth centuries in Eastern Europe as a reaction to Talmudic intellectualism. It was most popular in Poland and Russia and had a smaller following in Lithuania where its opponents, known as mitnagdim, were in the majority

Kashrut: matters related to the provision of kosher, or ritually fit, foodstuffs

Midrash: Rabbinic legends and lore

Mishna: Jewish law code, compiled in the second century, from oral traditions

Sephardim: Jews of Spanish and Portuguese origin

Shochet: religious functionary trained in shechita, the method of conducting slaughter according to religious law

Shul: popular Yiddish expression for synagogue

Talmud: compilation of the Mishna, and its commentary the Gemara, into a major compendium of Jewish literature containing both legal and narrative elements as well as the complete Rabbinic view of life

Yeshiva: centre for advanced Jewish studies. Its principal is known as the Rosh Yeshiva

Bibliography

I. UNIVERSITY AND COLLEGE RECORDS

1. *University of Glasgow, Archives*

    Matriculation Slips, Medical Faculty, 1895-1945
    Graduation Albums of the University of Glasgow
    List of Medical Students at the University of Glasgow 1800-1850
    Matriculation Albums, Anderson's College, Glasgow
    Minutes of the Medical Faculty of St. Mungo's College 1914-1941
    Minutes of the Faculty of Medicine, University of Glasgow 1925-1941
    Minutes of the Senate, University of Glasgow, 1787, 1831, 1928-1942
    Minute Book of Anderson's College Medical School, 1908-1945
    List of Residents of the Western Infirmary, Glasgow, 1900-1945
    List of Residents of the Glasgow Royal Infirmary, 1900-1945
    Glasgow Royal Infirmary: Annual Reports, 1900-1945
    Glasgow Royal Infirmary: Minutes of Meetings of Managers and Committee, 1933
    Gartnavel Royal Hospital, Glasgow: Dr. A. MacNiven File, 'Austrian Psychoanalysts'
    Records of the Lansdowne Clinic, 1935-1945

2. *Royal College of Physicians and Surgeons of Glasgow, Library*

    Licentiates of the Faculty of Physicians and Surgeons of Glasgow

3. *Glasgow University Library*

    Glasgow University Prize Lists 1830-1860

4. *University of Edinburgh, Medical Faculty*

    Minutes of the Faculty of Medicine, 1925-1939

5. *Edinburgh University Library, Special Collections*

    Minutes of the Senate 1779
    Matriculation Index, Medical Faculty 1760-1859
    Graduation Albums of the University of Edinburgh

6. *Royal College of Surgeons of Edinburgh, Library*

   Minute Book of the Education Committee and Board of Management of the Medical School of the Royal Colleges, Edinburgh 1924-1942
   Minute Book of the Governing Board of the School of Medicine of the Royal Colleges, Edinburgh, Vol. III, (1928-1945)
   Examination Slips, Final Examinations, Triple Qualification Board, 1933-1945
   Minutes of the Admission Committee of the Medical School of the Royal Colleges, Edinburgh 1933-1945

7. *University of Aberdeen, King's College Library*

   Minute Book of the Medical Faculty, Aberdeen University 1925-1940
   Minutes of Senatus Academicus, Aberdeen University, Vols. X-XII
   Graduation Albums of the University of Aberdeen.

8. *University of St. Andrews Library*

   Senate Minutes of the University of St. Andrews 1928-1929
   Graduation Albums of the University of St. Andrews

9. *King's College, London, Library*

   Delegacy Minutes

10. *University of Liverpool, Archives*

    Minutes of the Faculty of Medicine, University of Liverpool 1919-1940

11. *University of Leeds, Archives*

    Minutes of the Faculty of Medicine

II. OTHER UNPUBLISHED RECORDS

1. *Public Record Office, Kew, London*

   Home Office: registered correspondence on Jewish refugees and admittance of foreign doctors and medical students, 1933-1942 H045/15882/666764
   Foreign Office: political correspondence files (FO371) 1933-1945

2. *Bodleian Library, Oxford*

   Minutes and Records of the Society for the Protection of Science and Learning

3. *Mitchell Library, Glasgow*

   Strathclyde Regional Archives: Minute Books of the Parochial West Cadder, 1828-1866

4. *Jewish Archive Centre, Garnethill Synagogue, Glasgow*

   Minute Books of the Garnethill Hebrew Congregation, 1858-1919
   Annual Report of School Committee, Garnethill Hebrew Congregation, 1909-1910

5. *Dumfries and Galloway Health Board, Archives*

   Annual Reports, Crichton Royal Hospital, 1939-1950

6. *Jewish Welfare Board, London*

   Annual Reports of the Jewish Board of Guardians, London 1862-1866

III. PERIODICALS AND YEAR BOOKS

(a) Jewish

1. Jewish Echo 1928-
2. Jewish Chronicle 1878-
3. American Jewish Year Book 1918/9-1948/9
4. Jewish Year Book 1896-
5. Glasgow Jewish Year Books 1937/8-1938/9
6. Hashanah, Scottish Jewish Year Books 1955/6-1957/8
7. Transactions and Miscellanies of the Jewish Historical Society of England

(b) Medical

1. British Medical Journal 1930-1940
2. The Lancet 1930-1940
3. Journal of the American Medical Association 1930-1950
4. Surgeons' Hall Journal, the journal of the Medical School of the Royal Colleges of Edinburgh
5. Lister Journal, the journal of the extra-mural colleges of medicine in Glasgow 1939-1941
6. Medical Directory 1856-1945
7. Medical Register 1856-1945
8. Edinburgh Medical Journal 1891
9. Minutes of the General Medical Council, 1929 (Vol. LXVI)-1941 (Vol. LXXVIII)
10. Medical and Dental Students' Register (Lists of medical and dental students registered annually) 1920-1939

(c) Others

1. Post Office Directories for Glasgow 1850-1914
2. Post Office Directories for Edinburgh 1825-1835
3. Gentleman's Magazine and Historical Chronicle 1818-1825

IV. REFERENCE BOOKS

1. *Encyclopaedia Judaica* (Jerusalem 1972) 16 volumes
2. *The Jewish Encyclopaedia* (New York 1925) 12 volumes
3. Cecil Roth, *Magna Bibliotheca Anglo-Judaica* (1937)
4. Ruth Lehmann, *Anglo-Jewish Bibliography* (1973)
5. G. A. Lindeboom, *Dutch Medical Biography: A Biographical Dictionary of Dutch Physicians and Surgeons 1475-1975* (Amsterdam 1984)
6. *Dictionary of National Biography* (Oxford 1917)
7. *Universal Jewish Encyclopaedia* (New York 1943) 10 volumes
8. William Munk, *Roll of the Members of the Royal College of Physicians of London* (1978) 3 volumes
9. G. H. Brown, *Munk's Roll, Volume IV, Lives of the Fellows of the Royal College of Physicians of London* (1955)
10. *Britain and the Refugee Crisis 1933-1947* Imperial War Museum Oral History Recordings
11. Colonel William Johnston, *Roll of Commissioned Officers in the Medical Service of the British Army* (Aberdeen 1917)
12. D. G. Crawford, *Roll of the Indian Medical Service 1615-1930,* (1930)

V. ARTICLES AND BOOKS

Adams, Walter, 'The Refugee Scholars of the 1930's' *The Political Quarterly* Vol. 39, No. 1 (1968)

Anderson, P. J., *Officers and Graduates of University and King's College, Aberdeen 1495-1860* II, (Aberdeen 1893)

Anderson, R. D., *Education and Opportunity in Victorian Scotland: Schools and Universities* (Oxford 1983)

Anderson, Robert, 'Secondary Schools and Scottish Society, *Past and Present* 109 (1985)

────'Education and Society in Modern Scotland—A Comparative Perspective', *History of Education Quarterly* 25 (1985)

Andrade, J. A. P. M., *A Record of the Jews on Jamaica* (Kingston 1941)

Aronsfeld, C. C., 'German Jews in Dundee' *Jewish Chronicle* 20.11.1953

Ballon, Harry C., 'Aaron Hart David M.D.', *Canadian Medical Association Journal*, 1962 Vol. 86

Barnett, Richard, 'Dr. Jacob de Castro Sarmento and Sephardim in Medical Practice in Eighteenth Century London' *TJHSE*, XXVII (1982)

Benas, B. L., *Records of Jews in Liverpool*, (Liverpool 1900)

Bermant, Chaim, 'Anatomy of Glasgow' in *Explorations* ed. B. Mindlin and C. Bermant, (1967)
—— *Coming Home* (1976)
—— *The Jews* (1977)
—— *Troubled Eden* (1969)
Beveridge, Lord, *A Defence of Free Learning* (1959)
Bloch, Harry, 'The Berlin Correspondence in the JAMA During the Hitler Regime', *Bulletin of the History of Medicine* (1973)
Block, Geoffrey D. M. 'Jewish Students at the Universities of Great Britain and Ireland—excluding London 1936-1939, *Sociological Review* 34 1942
—— and Schwab, Harry, 'A Survey of Jewish Students at the British Universities', *Jewish Year Book* (1938)
Bloomgarden, Lawrence, '*A Preliminary Analysis of Discrimination against Jewish Applications to Medical School in New York State*', mimeographed and published privately by the American Jewish Committee (1952)
Bowers, John Z., 'The Influence of Edinburgh on American Medicine', in Gordon MacLachlan, (ed.) *Medical Education and Medical Care: A Scottish American Symposium* (1977)
Brock, Helen, 'Scotland and American Medicine', in William Brock, *Scotus Americanus* (Edinburgh 1982)
Brown, P. S., 'Herbalists and Medical Botanists in Mid-Nineteenth Century Britain with Special Reference to Bristol *Medical History* 26 1982
Burrows, Edmund H., *A History of Medicine in South Africa*, (Capetown 1958)
Camp, John, *The Healers Art* (1978)
Cant, R. G., *The University of St. Andrews*, (Edinburgh 1946)
Chitnis, Anand C., *The Scottish Enlightenment*, (1986)
Cohn-Zedek, Rev. D., *Asher Asher*, (1916) in Hebrew, bound with Asher Asher, *Collected Writings*
Collier, Adam, 'Social Origins of a Sample of Entrants to Glasgow University', *Sociological Review*, Vol. XXX (1938)
Collins, Kenneth, 'Angus MacNiven and the Austrian Psychoanalysts' *Glasgow Medicine* Vol. 2, No. 5 (1956)
—— 'Asher Asher, Doctor of the Poor' *Glasgow Medicine*, 2 (1984)
—— 'Quack Medicines in the Glasgow Advertiser 1798' *Scottish Medicine*, 3 (1983)
Comrie, J. D., *History of Scottish Medicine* 1 (1932)
Cooke, A. M., *A History of the Royal College of Physicians of London*, (Oxford 1972)
Coutts, James, *A History of the University of Glasgow* (Glasgow 1909)
Craig, W. S., *History of the Royal College of Physicians of Edinburgh* (Oxford 1976)
Crawford, D. G., *History of the Indian Medical Service*, (1934) 2 Vols.
Daiches, David, *Glasgow* (1977)
Daiches, David, *Two Worlds: An Edinburgh Jewish Childhood* (Sussex 1971)
Davie, George E., *The Democratic Intellect: Scotland and her Universities in the Nineteenth Century* (1964)
Duffy, John, *The Healers* (University of Illinois 1979)
Elzas, Bernard, *The Jews of South Carolina* (Philadelphia 1905)
Engel, Desider, *Pages of a Surgeon's Diary* (Jerusalem 1984)
Findlay, Ian R., *Education in Scotland* (Newton Abbot 1973)

Finestein, Israel, 'Anglo-Jewish Opinion During the Struggle for Emancipation 1828-1858' *TJHSE*, XX (1964)
Flexner, A., *Medical Education in the United States and Canada* (New York 1910)
Franklin, A. E., *Records of the Franklin Family* (1935)
Friedlander, Dr. M., 'Glasgow Jewish Education: A Survey of Activities', *Glasgow Jewish Year Book* (1937)
Freidenwald, Harry, *The Jews and Medicine* (Baltimore 1944) 3 Vols.
Gartner, Lloyd P., *The Jewish Immigrant in England 1870-1914* (1973)
Gillman, Peter and Leni, *Collar the Lot: How Britain Interned and Expelled its Wartime Refugees* (1980)
Girdwood, Ronald, 'Edinburgh in the History of Medicine' in Gordon MacLachlan (ed.) *Medical Education and Medical Care: A Scottish American Symposium* (1977)
Glasgow Herald 2.11.1917
Glazer, Nathan, 'Social Characteristics of American Jews 1654-1954' *American Jewish Year Book* Vol. 56, (1955)
Goldberg, Jacob A., 'Jews in the Medical Profession' *Jewish Social Studies* Vol. 1, (1939)
—— 'Jews in Medicine', *Medical Economics* March 1940
Goldman, L. M., *Jews in Victoria in the 19th Century* (Melbourne 1954)
Grant, W. Horseley, *Russian Medicine* (New York 1937)
Hamilton, David, *The Healers* (Edinburgh 1982)
Hearst, E., The attitudes of the popular press to the admission of the foreign doctors is considered in 'A Brain Gain Rejected', *Weiner Library Bulletin* Vol. XIX (1965)
Heaton, J. H., *Australian Dictionary of Dates* (Sydney 1879)
Herrman, Louis, *History of the Jews in South Africa* (Cape Town 1935)
Honigsbaum, Frank, *The Division in British Medicine* (1979)
Hook, Andrew, *Scotland and America* (Glasgow 1975)
Horn, D. B., *A Short History of the University of Edinburgh 1556-1889* (Edinburgh 1967)
Howe, Irving, *The Immigrant Jews of New York* (1976)
Hyamson, A. M., *The Sephardim of England* (1951)
Hyman, Louis, *The Jews of Ireland to 1910* (Shannon 1972)
Illingworth, Sir Charles, *University Stateman: Sir Hector Hetherington* (Glasgow 1971)
Innes-Smith, R. W., *English Speaking Students at the University of Leyden* (Edinburgh 1932)
Jacobs, Montague, 'Our Community and its Institutions, *Glasgow Jewish Year Book* (1937)
Jakobovits, Immanuel, *Jewish Medical Ethics* (New York 1967)
—— *Journal of a Rabbi* (1967)
Jarcho, Saul, 'Medical Education in the United States 1910-1956' *Journal of the Mount Sinai Hospital* Vol. XXXVI, No. 4
Kagan, Solomon R., *The Jewish Contribution to Medicine in America* (Boston 1939)
Kingdon, Frank, 'Discrimination in the Medical Colleges', *The American Mercury* Vol. LXI, No. 262
Kolmel, Rayner, 'Problems of Settlement: German Jewish Refugees in Scotland', *Exile in Great Britain: Refugees from Hitler's Germany*, Gerhard Hirschfeld (editor) (New Jersey 1984)

Kosmin, Barry, 'Localism and Pluralism in Jewry 1900-1980' *TJHSE*, Vol. XXVIII (1984)
Lamb, Margaret, 'The Medical Profession' in Olive Checkland and Margaret Lamb, *Health Care as Social History: The Glasgow Case* (Aberdeen 1982)
Levin, Salmond, 'Origins of the Jews' Free School', *TJHSE* (1959) Vol. 19
Levy, A., 'The Early Days of Glasgow Jewry', *Hashanah 1955-1956* (Glasgow 1955)
―― *The Origins of Scottish Jewry* (1958)
Lewis, Aubrey, 'William Mayer-Gross: An Appreciation' *Psychological Medicine* (1977) Vol. 7
Lipman, V. D. (ed.) *Three Centuries of Anglo-Jewish History* (1961)
Major, Ralph H., *A History of Medicine* (Oxford 1954)
Mathew, W. M., 'The Origins and Occupations of Glasgow Students: 1740-1839, *Past and Present* XXXIII (1966)
Morrell, J. B., 'Medicine and Science in the Eighteenth Century', in Gordon Donaldson (ed.) *Four Centuries: Edinburgh University Life* (Edinburgh 1983)
Morton, Frederick, *The Rothschilds* (1962)
Newman, Charles, *The Evolution of Medical Education in the Nineteenth Century* (1957)
Oren, Dan, *Joining the Club: A History of the Jews and Yale*, (New Haven 1985)
Parry, Noel and Parry, Jose, *The Rise of the Medical Profession* (1976)
Petersen, M. Jeanne, *The Medical Profession in Mid Victorian London* (1978)
Phillips, Abel, *A History of the Origins of the First Jewish Community in Scotland-Edinburgh 1816* (Edinburgh 1979)
Picciotto, James, *Sketches of Anglo-Jewish History*, ed. Israel Finestein (1956)
Pollins, Harold, *Economic History of the Jews in England* (1982)
Preuss, Julius, *Biblical and Talmudic Medicine* trans. Fred Rosner (New York 1977)
Reznikoff, Charles, *The Jews of Charlestown* (Philadelphia 1950)
―― 'New Haven: the Jewish Community' *Commentary* Vol. I (1947)
Rifkind, Lewis, (published by the Lewis Rifkind Memorial Book Committee in conjunction with Glasgow Poale Zion) n.d.
Risse, Guenter B., *Hospital Life in the Enlightenment Scotland: Care and Teaching at the Royal Infirmary of Edinburgh* (Cambridge 1986)
Roger, Ella Hill Burton, *Aberdeen Doctors at Home and Abroad* (Edinburgh 1893)
Ronder, Jack, *The Lost Tribe* (1978)
Rosenberg, Charles E., ed. *Healing and History: Essays for George Rosen* (1979)
Rosner, Fred, *Medicine in the Bible and Talmud* (New York 1977)
Rostowski, J., *History of the Polish School of Medicine: University of Edinburgh* (University of Edinburgh 1955)
Roth, Cecil, *A History of the Marranos* (Philadelphia 1932)
―― *The Jews in the English Universities* Miscellanies of the *JHSE* IV (1942)
―― *Rise of Provincial Jewry* (1950)
―― *The History of the Great Synagogue* (1950)
Rothstein, William G., *American Physicians in the Nineteenth Century* (Baltimore 1872)
Rubens, Alfred, 'Portrait of Anglo-Jewry' *TJHSE* (1959) Vol. XIX
Ruppin, Arthur, *Jews in the Modern World* (1934)
Sack, B. G., *History of the Jews in Canada* Vol. I (Montreal 1945)
Samuel, Edgar R., 'Anglo-Jewish Notaries and Scriveners', *TJHSE* (1953) Vol. XVII
―― 'Dr. Meyer Schomberg's Attack on the Jews of London', *TJHSE* (1964) Vol. XX

Sanderson, Michael, (ed.) *The Universities in the Nineteenth Century* (1975)
Schomberg, Meyer, 'Emunat Omen' (trans. Harold Levy), *TJHSE* (1964) Vol. XX
Shapin, Stephen, 'The Audience for Scottish Science', *Hist. Sci* XII (1974)
Shapiro, Alfred L., 'Racial Discrimination in Medicine' *Jewish Social Studies* Vol. 10, April 1948
Sherman, A. J., *Island Refuge: Britain and the Refugees from the Third Reich* (1973)
Sigerst, Henry E., 'Trends in Modern Education: A Program for a New Medical School', *Bulletin of the History of Medicine* Vol. IX (Baltimore 1941)
Silbermann, Charles, *A Certain People*, (New York 1985)
Skinnider, Sister Martha, 'Catholic Elementary Education in Glasgow: 1818-1919' in T. R. Bone (ed.) *Scottish Education: 1872-1939* (1967)
Smith, A. H. T., 'Medical Education at Oxford and Cambridge prior to 1850' in F. N. L. Poynter, *The Evolution of Medical Education in Britain* (1966)
Smout, T. C., *A Century of the Scottish People* (1986)
―― *A History of the Scottish People: 1560-1830* (1969)
Steinberg, Stephen, 'How Jewish Quotas Began', *Commentary* Vol. 52 September 1971
Stevens, Austin, *The Dispossessed* (1975)
Synott, Marcia Graham, *The Half-Opened Door: Discrimination and Admissions at Harvard, Yale and Princeton 1900-1970* (Westport 1979)
Tait, Allan C., *Review of Clinical Services (at Crichton Royal)*
Templewood, Lord (Sir Samuel Hoare), *Nine Troubled Years* (1954)
Thomson, C. J. S., *The Quacks of Old London* (1928)
Underwood, E. Ashworth, *Boerhaave's Men at Leyden and After* (Edinburgh 1977)
Watson, Francis, *Dawson of Penn* (1950)
Weschler, Harold S., *The Qualified Student: A History of Selective College Admission in America* (New York 1977)
Weidman, Jerome, 'May 27, 1939—Royal Bank of Scotland, St. Andrews Square, Edinburgh, Scotland—$50' *Letter of Credit* (New York 1940)
Williams, Bill, *The Making of Manchester Jewry 1740-1875* (Manchester 1985)
―― The Anti-Semitism of Tolerance: Middle-Class Manchester and the Jews 1870-1900' in A. J. Kidd and K. W. Roberts, eds., *City, Class and Culture: Studies of Cultural Production and Social Policy in Victorian Manchester* (Manchester 1985)
Winter, J., *Journal of Contemporary History* (15) 2 (1980)
Withers, Charles J., 'Kirk, Club and Culture Change: Gaelic chapels, Highland Societies and the urban Gaelic sub-culture in Eighteenth Century Scotland' *Social History* Vol. 10 No.2 (1985)
White, Jerry, *Rothschild Buildings* (1980)
Wolf, Lucien, *Essays in Jewish History* (1934)
Wright, Samson, 'Our Colleagues in Austria', letter, *Lancet* 9.4.1938
Young, Douglas, *St. Andrews* (1969)

Index

Abenheimer, Karl, 148
Aberdeen, Jewish community in, 58, 74, 75, 87
Aberdeen University, 15, 17, 24, 34, 35, 42, 165
    American medical students at, 114
    refugee students at, 146
    (*see also* Marischal College and King's college)
Academic Assistance Council, *see* Society for the Protection of Science and Learning
Adolphus, Edwin, 43, 163
Adolphus, Sir Javob, 37, 41, 163
Alberga, Marilyn, 48
Aliens Act (1905), 59
America, students from, (1748-1830), 16-17, 44
Amsterdam, 10, 33
Anderson's College Medical School, Glasgow, 28, 117, 146
Anglicisation, 12, 77, 78, 94
anti-alien agitation, 143
anti-semitism, 84-86
Arama, Isaac, 2
Asaph Ha-Rofe, 3
Ashenheim, Charles, 42, 43, 49, 51, 163
Ashenheim, Louis, 42, 43, 49, 51, 163, 164
Asher, Asher, 33, 51-54
Avigdor, Abraham, 8
Axelrod, Julius, 105
Ayr, Jewish community in, 75

Baruh, Daniel, 37, 164
Basel, Church Council of, 7
Belinfante, Simon, 42, 164, 165
Ben Sira, 1
Bennet, Simon Harry, 85
Bernstein, Meyer, 43, 165
Beveridge, Sir William, 141

Bevis Marks, (Congregation of Spanish and Portuguese Jews, London), 9, 33-35, 51, 167, 173, 174, 178
ibn Bikhlarish, Jonah, 3
Boerhaave, Herman, 18
Bravo, David, 43, 49, 165
Bravo, Moses, 43, 49, 165
British Medical Association, xvii, 134, 135, 143, 144, 148, 168, 177
Brodum, William, 37, 38, 40, 165

Cambridge, University of, 11, 13, 15, 18, 20, 23, 34
Cardozo, Samuel, 37, 165, 166
Carnegie Trust, 28, 29, 82, 89, 160
Carstares, William, 16
de Castro, Joao Periera, 43
de Castro, Miguel Caetano, 43, 167
Charteris, Frank, 114
City College New York, 100, 107, 108, 114
Cohen, David, 37, 166
Cohen, Douglas, 43, 51, 166
Cohen, Marx, 47
Cohen, Tobias, 8
Columbia University, 100-102, 107, 108
Cornell University, 106, 108
Cosgrove, Rev. Dr. I. K., 69
de la Cour, Philip, 41, 167, 176
Cullen, William, 22, 23, 43
Crichton Royal, Dumfries, 148
da Cunha, Joseph, 37, 166

Daiches, Rabbi Salis, 66, 68, 69, 125
Dalry Hebrew Congregation, Edinburgh, 60
Darragh, William, 107
David, Aaron Hart, 43, 50, 166
Davis, Maurice, 42, 51, 168
Dawson of Penn, Lord, xvii, 134-136
Donnolo, Shabbetai, 7
Dukes Place Synagogue, 51

INDEX

Dundee, Jewish community in, 58, 74, 75, 87
Dunfermline, Jewish Community in, 75

Ecclesiasticus, 1
Edinburgh, 24
Edinburgh, American medical students and the Jewish community, 123-127
    founding of Jewish community, 44, 57, 58, 59, 172
    growth of Jewish community, 65, 66
Edinburgh, University of, 15, 17, 19-21, 34, 37, 47, 51, 98
    American medical students, 111-114
    Jewish medical students and graduates, 88, 163-173, 176, 177
    Matriculation Album, 43
    Medical Faculty, 16, 23, 24, 26
    Polish School of Medicine, 153, 154
    refugee physicians and students at, 139
Emanuel, Leonard, 42, 168
Emergency Medical Services, 151
emigration, 42
employment, Jewish,
    in Edinburgh, 60
    in Glasgow, 61, 62, 74, 76-78
English medical schools, American students at, 119, 120

Falkirk, Jewish community in, 74, 75, 87
Fishbein, Morris, 106
Flexner Report, 101
Fraenkel, Henry, 43, 49, 168
Frankfurt-am-Oder, University of, 9
Franklin, Isaac Abraham, 50, 51

Garcia, Daniel, 37, 168
Garnethill Synagogue, Glasgow, 54, 55, 60, 64, 65, 69, 81, 90, 95, 125, 171
General Medical Council, 109-111, 134, 151, 160
Glasgow Advertiser, see *Glasgow Herald*
Glasgow Hebrew Congregation, see Garnethill Synagogue
Glasgow Herald, 38-40, 167, 176
Glasgow, American medical students and the Jewish community, 123-7
    founding of Jewish community, 44, 47, 57-59

Gorbals Jewish community, 61, 65, 66, 70, 72, 74, 94
Jewish refugees from Germany, 59, 60
movement from Gorbals, 90, 91
new synagogues formed, 66
see also entries for individual organisations
Glasgow, University of, 15, 28, 98
    American medical students at, 111-113
    Medical Faculty, 19, 23, 24
    Jewish medical students and graduates, 87-89, 164, 170, 171, 173
    refugee physicians and students, 139
Goldsmith, Oliver, 20
Goodenough Report, 92, 120, 121
Goodman, Hyam, 85
Gavin, Frank, 103
Graham Street Synagogue, Edinburgh, 64, 66, 70
Great Synagogue, Glasgow, *see* South Portland Street Synagogue
Greenock, Jewish community in, 75
Gross, Reuben, 52, 168

Halevi, Judah, 3
Harris, Saul, 61, 85
Hart, Joel, 43, 47, 51, 168
Harvard University, 100
Hebra, *see* Bevis Marks
Henriques, Ernest, 48
Henriques, Horace Leslie Cohen, 48
Henriques, Joseph Gutteres, 43, 48, 169
Henriques, Moses Nunes, 43, 48, 169
Herxheimer, Herbert, 154, 156, 157
Herz, Marcus, and Maimonides' Oath, 6
Hetherington, Sir Hector, 146
Hoare, Sir Samuel, 143, 144, 152

in absentia, degrees awarded, 24, 25, 35, 42
Iffla, Solomon, 42, 49, 169
Indian Medical Service, 42, 170, 177
Inquisition, 1, 35, 174
institutional care, Jewish, 64
internment,
    First World War, 65
    Second World War, 151, 152
Inverness, Jewish community in, 75, 85

Irvine, Sir James, 114, 115
Israeli, Isaac, 3, 7

Jamaica, Jewish students and doctors from, 48-50, 163, 164, 167, 169, 173, 177
Jarcho, Saul, 103
Jewish Board of Glasgow, 59, 61, 62, 85, 95, 125
Jewish Board of Guardians, London, 53, 59n, 164
Jewish Echo, Glasgow, 74, 124
Jewish Friendly Societies, 62, 64, 67, 95
Jewish Institute, Glasgow, 64
Jewish Medical Emergency Association, 134, 141
Jewish Representative Council, Glasgow, 65, 70
Jewish Students' Society,
  Glasgow, 76, 77, 83
  Edinburgh, 76, 77, 83
Jewish Welfare Clinic and Dispensary, Glasgow, 62, 85
Jewish women in medicine, 86, 87
Joseph, Joseph Marcus, 52, 170
Joseph, Laurence, 47, 52, 170

King's College, Aberdeen, 24, 34, 37, 41, 172-174
Kraemer, William, 151
Kramrisch, Jacob, 61

lad o' pairts, 20
Lara, Benjamin, 35, 37, 41, 43, 51, 170
Laurence, Joseph, *see* Laurence Joseph
Lazarus, Samuel, 92
Leiden, University of, 10, 16, 18, 20, 167
Leo, Luis, 38, 41, 171
de Leon, Hananel, 43, 48, 51, 167
de Leon, Solomon, 35, 43, 48, 51, 167
Levenston family, medical botanists, 54, 55
Levenston, Samuel, 54, 55, 81, 171
Levy, Michael, 43, 49, 171
Lewisohn, Gumpertz, 37, 171
Lion, Heyman, 41, 43, 51, 172
Lipetz, Sam, 92, 93
Lipsey, Jacob, 95
Lowell, A. Lawrence, 100
Lurie, Rabbi Jacob David, 93-95
Lurie, Mendel, 95
Lyon, Benjamin, 37

MacGowan, Peter K., 148, 155
MacNiven, Angus, 148, 155
Maimonides, Moses (Rambam), 1, 3, 4, 7, 54
Mann (Teitlemann), Meyer, T., 82, 85, 86, 94
Marischal College, Aberdeen, 24, 34, 35, 37, 40, 41, 44, 163, 167, 170-175, 177, 178
Marranos, 10, 33
Mayer-Gross, William, 148, 155
Medical Practitioners' Union, 134, 143, 144, 152
Mendes da Costa, A. R. (Abraham Raphael), 43, 44, 172
Mendes da Costa, Hananel, 43, 172
Mennons, John, 40
Meyer, John, 41, 172
Michaelson, Isaac Chesar, 92
missionaries, 62
Montefiore, Judah Israel, 35, 37, 49, 173
Montefiore, Sir Moses, 169, 173
Montpellier, 8, 9
Montreal, 50, 166
Morris, Professor Noah, 85, 86, 94
Myers, Joseph Hart, 35, 41, 43-47, 173, 174
Myers, Levi, 43, 47, 52, 173, 174

New York University, 100, 106, 114

Orr, John, 118, 119, 127, 129, 137, 139, 140, 155
Oxford, University of, 11, 13, 15, 18, 20, 23, 34

Pacifico, Emanuel de Asher, 35, 37, 174
Padua, University of, 8
Parliament (Scots), 15, 19
Pereira, Jonathan, 47
Phillips, Rev. E. P., 69
Pinkerton, Myre Conrad, 96
Poland, pre-war Jewish community, 153
Polish School of Medicine, *see* Edinburgh University
Pope Julius, 8
Preuss, Julius, 2

Rambam, *see* Maimonides
Rappleye, Willard. C., 109, 118, 129
religious education, Glasgow Jewish, 70, 71-73

INDEX

religious leadership, Jewish, 69
religious observance, Jewish, 68, 69
religious tests, (Scotland), 19-20, 44
Rifkind, Lewis, 76, 152
Rodman, J. S., 111
Rongy, A. I., 104
Rosen, George, 106
Roth, Cecil, 11
Royal College (Faculty) of Physicians and Surgeons of Glasgow, 15, 23
Royal Colleges of Edinburgh, Medical School of, 28, 112, 127-129
    American medical students at, 118
Royal Infirmary, Edinburgh, 22, 84, 130
Royal Infirmary, Glasgow, 23, 28, 84, 139, 155
    refugee physicians at, 137
Royal Medical Society, Edinburgh, 20, 168, 172
Rush, Benjamin, 17
Rypins, Harold, 102-104, 128

St. Andrews, Univeristy of, 15, 17, 24, 25, 35, 83, 98, 128, 164
    American medical students at, 114
St. Mungo's School of Medicine, Glasgow, 28, 146
    American medical students at, 114, 117, 127
    refugee physicians at, 137
Salerno, 7, 8
Samuel, Mar, 2
Sarmento, Jacob de Castro, 34, 35, 37, 44, 174
Schomberg, Meyer, 41, 174, 175
Schomberg, Ralph, 35, 37, 41, 175
Schwitella, A. M., 103
Scotland, Church of, 18
Sequira, Joseph, 41, 176
Sharman, Albert, 92

Sigerst, Henry, 103
Slater, Oscar, 70
Smith, Adam, 22, 25
Society for the Protection of Science and Learning, 141, 142, 147
Solomon, Abraham, 37, 176
Solomon, Samuel, 37, 40, 176
South Africa, Jewish students from, 49, 76
South Portland Street Synagogue, Glasgow, 65
Steinschneider, Moritz, 8
Stengel, Erwin, 148, 151, 155
Stern, Moritz, 43, 48, 50, 177

transmigrants, 60, 61
Triple Qualification Board, 120, 135, 136, 139, 140, 144, 146, 154, 155, 161

University College, Dundee, 27
University College, London, 11-13
Universities Test Act (1871), 11

Victoria Infirmary, Glasgow, 137

Wallich, George Charles, 37, 43, 177
Wallich, Nathaniel, 35, 37, 177
Wessels, Hart, 40, 41
Western Infirmary, Glasgow, 28, 84, 137
Winternitz, Milton Charles, 107

Yale University, 107

Zappfe, A., 111, 112
Zarfati, Rabbi Samuel, 8
Zeigler, Alexander, 42, 51
Zeigler, William, 178
Zionism, Glasgow, 73, 76, 77, 152

89041 3284
24/1/89
PERGAMON

Diploma awarded to David Collins by the Triple Qualification Board, 1941.

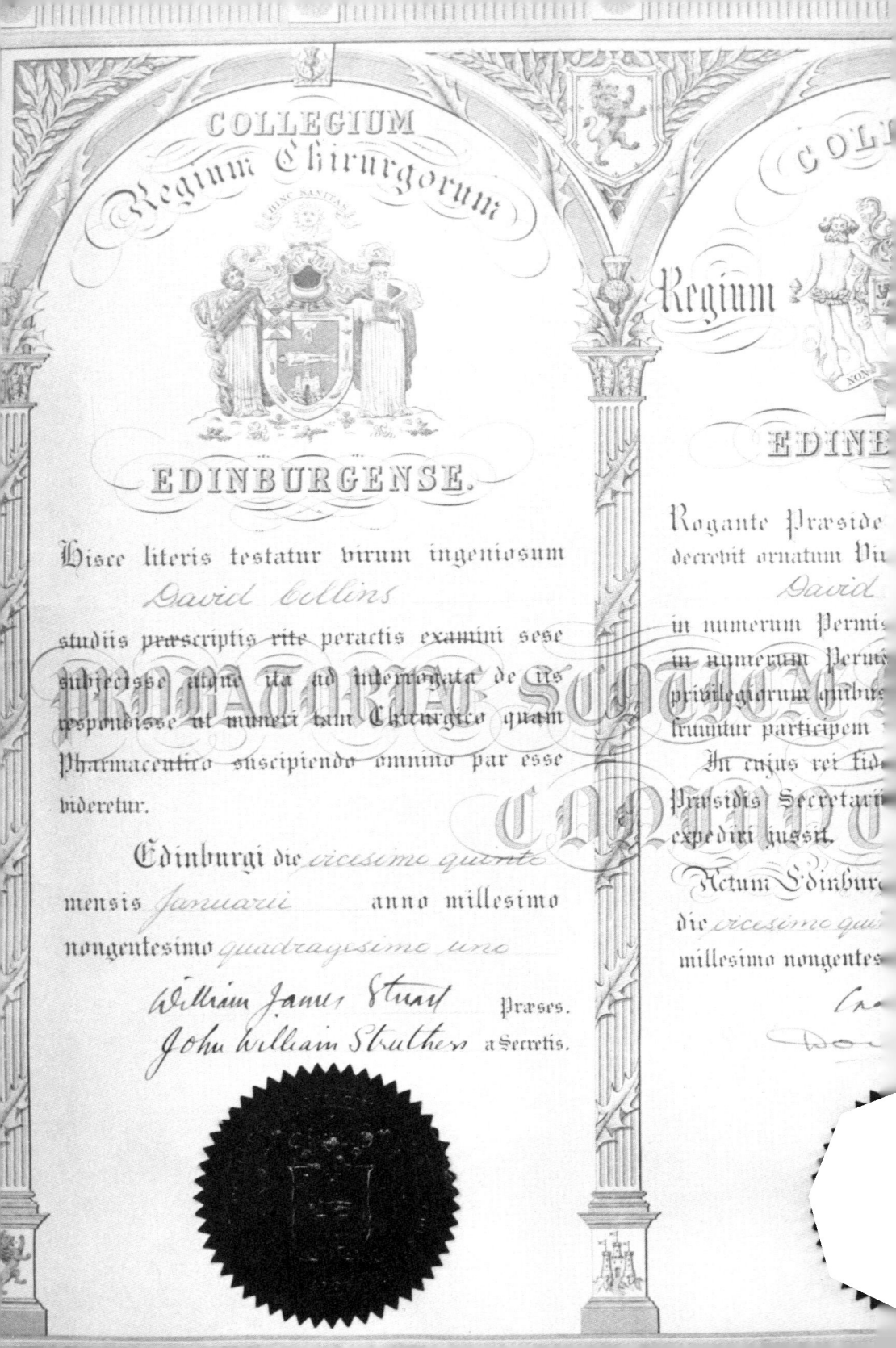